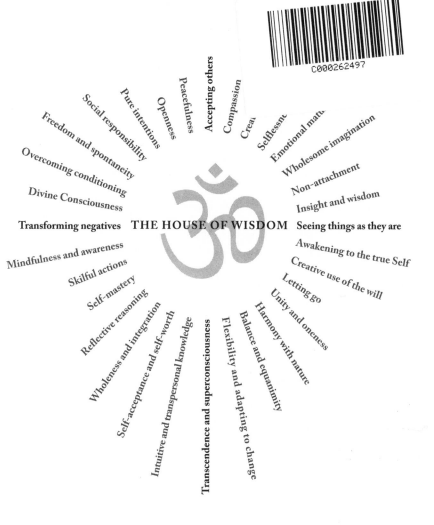

Accepting others
Compassion
Crea...
Selflessne...
Emotional matu...
Wholesome imagination
Non-attachment
Insight and wisdom

Peacefulness
Openness
Pure intentions
Social responsibility
Freedom and spontaneity
Overcoming conditioning
Divine Consciousness

Transforming negatives   **THE HOUSE OF WISDOM**   Seeing things as they are

Awakening to the true Self
Creative use of the will
Letting go
Unity and oneness
Harmony with nature
Balance and equanimity
Flexibility and adapting to change

Mindfulness and awareness
Skilful actions
Self-mastery
Reflective reasoning
Wholeness and integration
Self-acceptance and self-worth
Intuitive and transpersonal knowledge
Transcendence and superconsciousness

Also by the authors

Swami Dharmananda Saraswati Maharaj

Breath of Life: Breathing for Health, Vitality and Meditation

The Dynamic Body: Movements for Health, Vitality and Holistic Living (forthcoming)

Santoshan with Glyn Edwards

Tune in to your Spiritual Potential

Unleash your Spiritual Power and Grow: Reflect and Learn to Trust the Power Within

THE HOUSE
OF WISDOM

Yoga Spirituality of the East and West

Swami Dharmānanda
and Santoshan

Foreword by
Glyn Edwards

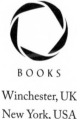

BOOKS

Winchester, UK
New York, USA

First published by O Books, 2007
O Books is an imprint of John Hunt Publishing Ltd.
The Bothy, Deershot Lodge,
Park Lane, Ropley,
Hants, SO24 0BE, UK
office@o-books.net
www.o-books.net

Distribution in:

UK and Europe
Orca Book Services
orders@orcabookservices.co.uk
Tel: 01202 665432 Fax: 01202 666219 Int. code (44)

USA and Canada
NBN
custserv@nbnbooks.com
Tel: 1 800 462 6420 Fax: 1 800 338 4550

Australia and New Zealand
Brumby Books
sales@brumbybooks.com.au
Tel: 61 3 9761 5535 Fax: 61 3 9761 7095

Far East (offices in Singapore, Thailand, Hong Kong, Taiwan)
Pansing Distribution Pte Ltd
kemal@pansing.com
Tel: 65 6319 9939 Fax: 65 6462 5761

South Africa
Alternative Books
altbook@peterhyde.co.za
Tel: 021 447 5300 Fax: 021 447 1430

Yoga is union; it is universal.
Just as the rays of the sun touch all beings,
so the Divine Light of all knowledge is there for us all.
Let us share in this Divine universal knowledge
with love and gratitude.
SWAMI DHARMANANDA

The path of universal wisdom leads to
embracing all as a spiritual whole and
overcoming the boundaries between ourselves and others.
It is an ever-evolving process of opening our hearts,
healing our wounds, accepting our differences,
and awakening our individual sense of self
to richer fields of being and consciousness.
SANTOSHAN

Dedication
This book is dedicated to all teachers and students of the past and present, who have endeavoured to promote and live a universal spirituality.

Special Thanks
We wish to thank our friends who encouraged us to collaborate in the production of this book and helped in deciding its contents.

A special thanks goes to John Chapman, member of Thich Nhat Hanh's Order of Interbeing (Tiep Hien), and to Fleur Maule who kindly assisted us with the proof reading.

Swamiji wishes to give a personal thanks to Santoshan for his help in compiling her chapters, and also wishes to thank her teachers, particularly Paramahansa Satyananda Saraswati and Sri Trivadi Ramachandra for their deep wisdom and encouragement.

Contents

List of Illustrations and Charts

About the Authors

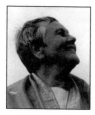

Swami Dharmananda Saraswati Maharaj is a member of the British Wheel of Yoga and the Spiritual Director of the Dharma Centre for Yoga, Spiritual Awareness and Healing. She became associated with the Bihar School of Yoga in 1973 and was later initiated as a sannyasin of the Saraswati Dasanami (order founded by Shankara) by Paramahansa Satyananda Saraswati. Her main spiritual teacher was Sri Trivadi Ramachandra (one-time secretary to Mahatma Gandhi).

She was given the task of promoting yogic teachings to lay people in the West. While deeply grounded in her own tradition, she has moved beyond religious boundaries to touch and benefit those from various faiths, including Christianity, Judaism, Jainism, Buddhism and Hinduism.

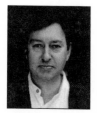

Santoshan (Stephen Wollaston) is the wisdom studies and creative adviser of the Gordon Higginson Fellowship for Integral Spirituality. He holds a degree in religious studies and a post graduate certificate in religious education from King's College London. He also studied graphic design at the London College of Printing and Psychosynthesis psychology and has a background as a musician.

His postgraduate studies focused on Critical Realist philosophy and holistic approaches in spiritual education. Additionally, the pragmatic approach of the historical Buddha, the teachings of Matthew Fox, Sri Aurobindo's Integral Yoga and Ken Wilber's stages of development have also influenced his current understanding.

Foreword

GLYN EDWARDS (DEVADASA)

It is pleasing to write a foreword to a book that explores the heart of spiritual wisdom. In every age there are people who possess a clear picture of the fundamentals of spirituality and provide us with profound insights for living life deeply. The authors often challenge us to reassess where we are now and our understanding of what spirituality entails. Their central message is one of compassion and unity, which involves realising our more creative and authentic natures, qualities and potentials. Above all, they urge us to dive deep into the depths of our being and realise our true Divinity and how to skilfully live by It.

Like many, I have been deeply touched and profoundly affected by Swamiji's presence and her common sense approach to spirituality. The radiance of her teachings gives hope during despair, direction in uncertainty and a greater understanding of the infinite possible potentials of who we truly are.

As much as the two authors share in common, Santoshan has taken a uniquely different route to Swamiji. His experience of many areas of development – educational, transpersonal, artistic and academic – has provided him with excellent personal insight into holistic and integral growth. In the understanding that Truth is inclusive and universal, both writers present a deep ecumenical approach to spirituality and a broad outlook on core developmental matters. They can both be considered as integral non-dualists, as they both view development as a process of including various disciplines, transforming the whole of ourselves and awakening to the One Supreme Reality that unites us all.

This book draws on a wealth of experience and presents it in a profoundly moving way. Guidance is given on a range of central topics, including integrating the spiritual into everyday life and facing difficulties on the path. Thoughts and observations put forward make inspiring connections between ancient wisdom and contemporary living. The opening part focuses on general themes, such as starting out on the journey, our many selves and problems that are frequently encountered. The second and fourth parts include many practical exercises. The third section looks closely at yogic wisdom, with crucial chapters on mantra and ways to the true Self. The knowledge shared in the appendices on three of the great traditions is for those who wish to be more informed about their depth, vibrancy and diversity.

Because of my early background as a Christian contemplative, my many years work as an intuitive, and a wide interest in yogic philosophy and practice, I was grateful for the bringing together of information in Appendix II, which puts forward a highly balanced view of how spirituality and psychic powers interrelate. Yet all the sections of this book are indispensable and, for me, the beating heart of this treasury of wisdom is the two chapters *Transformations in Development* and *Love is Only Part of it*, which show the authors writing at their most skilled about the essentials of spirituality.

In a time when the world is going through a difficult period in its history, books such as this offer practical advice about humankind's evolvement. In my view it is destined to become an important classic. I hope that its universal message falls on vast fields of fertile ground and will be shared by many.

Introduction

SANTOSHAN

There is frequently a price to pay for making headway into spiritual heartlands, but it is always worth the expense of any effort. The Thai Buddhist and meditation teacher Achaan Chah would tell students they hadn't meditated until they had wept. The Tibetan master Chogyam Trungpa would advise people that if they hadn't already started on the spiritual path it was best not to bother, as it was too difficult! Nonetheless, he would add that if they had started, it was best to continue.

There is a tendency to think of spiritual growth as just blissing-out or simply going with the flow of worldly life. Compared with doing some spiritual work these can seem like comfortable things to enjoy. But we will invariably not be happy doing them for long, as the call of our authentic Self will find ways of making itself known. However, as Achaan Chah and Trungpa remind us, the road is not always easy.

As parts of our old self and values are called into question we can encounter various stages of disenchantment. If we look at the Buddha's journey we see how a form of existential anxiety forced him to leave his luxurious palace and search for solutions to life's unsatisfactoriness. The teachings of the *Bhagavad Gita* start from the point of Arjuna's despondency, which lead him to numerous questions about the path he needs to take. There is an apt saying about preferring to be Socrates dissatisfied and searching for answers, than complacent and unaware of a spiritual way of life and living.

We need to ask ourselves if we are prepared to take up the challenge of change in order to discover a deeper meaning and purpose to life and the Ultimate Mystery of existence. We may make many false starts and take various wrong turns. We might encounter numerous stages of the dark night of the soul, where aspects of ourselves are refined in order to make our hearts and minds more open to Light.

The road to peace lies in seeing all these things as opportunities for learning and discovering our true nature. Every moment can be a time for growth, healing and transformation. When things fall apart and problems surface, we must ask ourselves what core issues lie behind them? What is the hidden creative potential to be found in life's difficulties? For all negatives are distortions of our authentic nature and the Ultimate Creativity that exists in the universe.

Wholeness is accomplished by embracing, integrating and balancing all areas, and coming to a maturity where we no longer keep different parts of ourselves in separate boxes. In Mahayana Buddhism they speak of the realisation of Nirvana being *samsara* and of *samsara* being Nirvana – a realisation that everyday life cannot be separated from spiritual understanding and living.

It is not possible to draw a clear line between the sacred and the profane, the spiritual and the secular, and to say that this is where one ends and the other begins. Any teaching that encourages a split between the two must surely be questioned, as it will lead us to seeing ourselves as separate from others. Yet we can talk of different levels of reality; of what is often seen as a 'two truths' existence: the Ultimate and the relative. But the truth is that everything is interwoven. The sacred is in the here and now. All is interrelated and "All life is Yoga", as Sri Aurobindo pointed out. An expanding spirituality includes the whole of existence and the whole of ourselves.

The road to lasting happiness lies in a higher reasoning and a compassionate life that relates to others, heals all wounds and connects with the world. To achieve this we have to search deeply into our hearts, overcome our limitations and learn how to contribute creatively to the welfare of humanity and life on Earth.

The path of the *Bhagavad Gita*, of various yogas, of the Buddha and of many Sufi and Christian contemplatives is a way of being fully present, participating in and awake to life. Solutions to life's entanglements do not lie in fighting against them, but in acceptance, seeing things as they are, in awakening to our original goodness and acting wisely in all situations.

If you have not done so already, I hope that the following pages will help you to embrace and motivate you to explore the richness of these ancient traditions, and to discover how they can still be as relevant and important today as ever.

I recently read about someone finding ancient grains of corn that were found in a two thousand year old Egyptian tomb. When the corn was planted, it grew. Although the early Egyptian culture has long-since disappeared and we have modern methods of turning corn into edible food, the grains are still living things, which can be cultivated and used with contemporary knowledge and understanding.

Before finishing this introduction I should say something about why this book has the sub-title *Yoga Spirituality of the East and West* and something about its contents. Firstly, yoga is no longer just an Eastern practice; it has been a part of Western culture for several decades. Secondly, like any living tradition, it is growing and changing to the needs of people in the world today and there are also Western teachers who have given it new perspectives. Lastly, as yoga can be interpreted to simply mean 'discipline' or 'practice', the West can be said to have its own forms of yoga, such as modern psychology, philosophy and numerous teachings on spirituality.

With this in mind, you will find that the following pages not only mention yoga in its traditional form, but also include teachings and insights from other traditions. Readers will notice that Swamiji and I have endeavoured to keep technical Sanskrit words to their minimum and have placed the majority of them in brackets for readers who are interested in knowing about them. There is also a glossary of key Sanskrit words at the back of the book. Overall we have aimed at writing in an accessible style in order to make the teachings and practices as comprehensible as possible. We hope that the following chapters will give you much food for thought on your spiritual journey and will encourage you to find and live your truth in daily life.

PART ONE
Reflections for Travellers

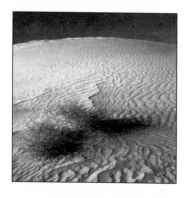

From the Centre of Divinity we begin,
to the Centre of Divinity we return.
SWAMI DHARMANANDA

To know ourselves is to realise the whole of who and what we are,
and the infinite creative potential within us.
SANTOSHAN

O seeker, know that the path to Truth is within you.
You are the traveller. Going happens by itself.
Coming happens to you, without you.
There is no arriving or leaving; nor is there any place;
nor is there a contained within a container.
Who is there to be with God? What is there other than God?
Who seeks and finds when there is none but God?
SHEIK BADRUDDIN

God is love and those that live in love live in God and God lives in them.
THE FIRST LETTER OF JOHN

Empty yourself of everything.
Let the mind rest at peace …
With an open mind, you will be open-hearted.
Being open-hearted, you will act royally.
Being royal, you will be at one with the Tao.
Being at one with the Tao is eternal.
TAO TE CHING

Arouse a heart of boundless kindness
for all things and all creatures
– upwards and downwards and across the world.
Unhindered, free of hate and enmity.
NIPATA SUTTA

Growth into the freedom of peace and silence is not the privilege of a chosen few.
It's the natural state of being for everyone.
VIMALA THAKAR

1

Beginning the Search

SWAMI DHARMANANDA

All is Brahma, All is Brahma!
What is worth saying
And what is not worth saying?
What is worth writing
And what is not worth writing?
PRASNA UPANISHAD

What can one say to spiritual travellers about the Divine and the spiritual life? What words can convey the vastness of yoga and the Supreme Union with God? What can be written that has not been written of the glory, the love, the compassion and the light of the Divine Lord and the Mother?

On the one hand I have to ask myself these questions as I put my pen to paper, while also reassuring myself that the Divine is forever revealing Itself in new acts of inspiration and invariably needs to be reflected upon in the light of current understanding.

The beginning of the journey

Explorers of the spiritual life take up various practices for different reasons. For some it may be about performing postures for their physical benefits and to make the body more supple and toned up. Others might seek therapeutic benefits through meditation or breathing exercises. Then there are those who look for wisdom and ethical guidance in the various philosophical schools of thought. Some have no specific reason and just start looking to see what spirituality is all about. Within the yoga traditions the practices are so diverse that they can cater for the various needs and motives of different spiritual explorers; for there is not just one way of beginning the journey to the ultimate knowledge of the Divine. Each and everyone will have their own discoveries to make. Even if some travel the same road together for a while, their individual experiences will be unique for each one of them.

Just as Jesus said, "In my Father's Kingdom there are many mansions", it is also recognised in the various yogic traditions that everyone has a special and unique path to follow – this is our *dharma*, our personal responsibility and way to God. If we follow our path in the light of our *dharma*, we will find the help we need for gaining knowledge of the spiritual life: "Seek and you shall find."

Sometimes we are glad to have the company as we travel on our journey. If our, or a companion's, load gets too heavy we can share our burdens for a while and help each other along the way. If we come to diversions on the path and decide to try different routes, we can part with the knowledge that we will eventually meet again, as all paths lead to the top of the mountain – the inner Sanctum.

We may discover the need for guides to show us the way, and to help us through the inevitable hazards and trouble spots, so that we do not get stranded or lose our way. We may, and more often than not we will, need some instructions to give us a deeper understanding and awareness of what the path entails. But we must choose our guides and teachers wisely and carefully if we wish to travel far on our journey. Compassion and universal love are the things to look for in the great masters of spirituality.

Sometimes we may have to change our guides or go on alone for a while. The hero or heroine on his or her quest for the Grail is sometimes used as a metaphor for this. It is a time that requires us to develop degrees of self-reliance and our own inner strength, intuition, insight and personal understanding in order to move forward in our development. It can be seen as a learning situation which teaches us about some of the essentials of spiritual growth.

Finding traces
The path may be difficult at times and beset with obstacles, but with perseverance we can attain an awareness of our relationship with

the Divine. We can look for inspiration and encouragement in the teachings of the great ones of the past. Jesus showed a way of living and acting in the world with compassionate understanding. His teachings have spread hope, spiritual light and knowledge of a life eternal.

In yogic teachings and texts, such as the *Bhagavad Gita* and *Srimad Bhagavatam*, various paths are mentioned. They recommend methods of conduct to be taken-up and outline numerous practices that can help us to find and manifest profound qualities of the Divine in our lives. The great wisdom traditions are the stepping-stones to inner knowledge which can teach us about awakening to a higher life and to our true spiritual existence.

If we are to work towards a realisation of our oneness with the Divine, then our spiritual practices should not be confined to the meditation or exercise room, but need to become an integral part of our being. Our practices should help us to discover and truly live by our Divinity in every moment. If we wish to be part of spreading this knowledge, then we must honour the teachings that can lead us to this awareness and recognise the omnipresent spark of the Divine in all, and all things in the Divine.

Upsets on the path

Sometimes we feel inadequate, especially when we are with others who appear to be more advanced in their learning or knowledge. We may even feel like failures when things do not go the way we expect them. But we need to remember that there are no failures in God's eyes. There is not one yardstick by which everyone is measured – the Divine has a place for everyone. We therefore have to have trust in the process of spiritual unfoldment and do the work that is needed for us to continue on our journey. A quotation comes to mind:

> *Water is for fish*
> *The air for men*
> *Natures differ,*
> *and needs with them.*
> *Hence the wise men of old*
> *Did not lay down*

One measure for all.
CHUANG TZU

It is in times of uncertainty and spiritual dryness that we need to persist with our spiritual practices, in order to unfold fresher insights about our relationship with the Divine, and to realise that even our worries and concerns are part of the growing process.

Opening and sharing along the way

True spirituality is about taking our practices into the world and sharing our gifts and wisdom with each other, as well as our joys and aspirations, and our sorrows and our pains, as there is nothing that is not part of this important journey. The work is like a kaleidoscope, the patterns and colours changing all the time. But we should realise that without change there is no growth – life is like this. And what is yoga but an embracing of life with Unity.

The teachings of yoga cover all aspects (the physical, the mental and the spiritual) and walks of life (householders, students and *sannyasis*). All things are ultimately woven together in the interactive dance of Shiva and Shakti (the cosmic creative rhythm of life), in the music of Krishna as he plays his flute and in the inspiration of Saraswati as she extols her teachings of wisdom. All things portray various aspects of One Reality, and are all bound together in the love, compassion, glory and light of the immanent and transcendent Divine Consciousness.

So let us then join Shiva and Shakti in the Dance of Life, sing to the music of Krishna's flute and chant the wisdom of the Divine with the Goddess Saraswati, as we continue our important journey of discovery.

Discovering different routes

Much has been said about the practices of postures, *pranayama* and meditation in yoga, but these are not the only paths. For many, spirituality and yoga might be about the cultivation of discerning wisdom, a devotional path, or a way of acting with pure and right intentions in the world. The answer to humankind's quest to 'know themselves' can be found in these various paths. Our innate wisdom can be discovered through them, which can then guide us further in our development.

Whatever route we take, it should bring about profound changes in our nature, in different levels of our being. These deeper changes can only take place with a disciplined application of the practices that we undertake, along with wholesome attitudes of mind that instil deep spiritual levels of awareness.

A revealing faith

An essential ingredient of the spiritual life is faith (termed 'shraddha' in Sanskrit). Faith can inspire things to happen; it can remove mountains and reveal the truth of who and what we are, why we are here and where we are going in our spiritual journey. It can also bring forth the power of inner healing by leading us to see life from greater perspectives and by helping us to let go of unskilful patterns of behaviour. Ultimately it is faith that keeps our faltering steps on the path of *dharma*. It is faith in the Divine Spirit that brings about an unfolding knowledge of our authentic Self and unites us with the Light of our True Being – what can be seen as the Supreme Awakening:

> *The man of faith who is devoted to spiritual knowledge and the practice of self-control gains wisdom. Having obtained wisdom, he gains supreme peace at once.*
> BHAGAVAD GITA

2

Expanding our Circle of Awareness

SANTOSHAN

*We are not only what we know of ourselves
but an immense more which we do not know;
our momentary personality is only a bubble
on the ocean of our existence.*
SRI AUROBINDO

A restrictive sense of our individual 'I', our individual sense of self, has long been seen as the chief cause of creating disenchantment. The great wisdom traditions tell us much about unhealthy conditioning which feeds self-centred drives, interests and desires, and how this hides our more authentic nature and our connection with the sacredness of all life.

The teachers of the ancient *Upanishads* remind us that spiritual growth should lead us from individual selfhood to realising our more universal selves and immerse us in the eternal reality of the true I-Consciousness – the One Interconnected Self that permeates everything and everyone.

A state of separateness
This limited sense of individual self is often termed 'the ego', which is not just about being ego-centric, but about how we see ourselves as separate from other life and cut off from greater levels of awareness.

If we look at this level of ourselves we will see that it comes with its own baggage, consisting mostly of images about us and our relationship with others that are not new or fresh, because they are filtered through old concepts that restrict our growth. But the news isn't all bad; there are other levels that are unitive, expansive and transcendent that can help us break-free from the limitations of the individual 'I'.

When we explore this level of ourselves we begin to see that we shape personalities around it, which we believe ourselves to truly be. We notice that we identify ourselves with being this or that type of person, with particular likes, dislikes and character traits. We might even deliberately build a false ideal image of ourselves to present to others (what Jung called the 'persona').

The problem is that we can waste so much energy in trying to keep these images of ourselves maintained and defended from anything we feel threatens us, that we end up losing sight of other realms of being.

Opening to greater possibilities

We find that spiritual practices, such as mindfulness and deep reflection, can help us to fully open ourselves to experience, cut through restrictive concepts of our ego and personality, and diminish desires about how we want things to be.

Contrary to what an unhealthy ego-personality might believe, no man or woman is an island. We all rely on others to survive and live healthily. The food we eat and the clothes we wear are usually the products of other people. We cannot live healthily without intimate relationships. We may restrictively extend this intimacy to only a few closest to us, but a genuinely creative and abundant life finds deep and meaningful relationships in all areas and cares and works towards the good of all people.

Authentic development leads us out of self-centredness to self-lessness where we realise our true relationship with life, and honour and respect the numerous ways in which we support one another. The Jewish philosopher Martin Buber wrote about experiencing the Divine in mutually affirming social interactions that overcome our separateness and awaken us to profound 'I-Thou' relationships with others (an experience of Divinity that is realised in healthy encounters with other people).

The volitional, creative and spiritual 'I'

Connected with the individual I-consciousness is our volitional self, the active personal will with its individual motivations. The will is the energy behind conscious activity and links with practices of karma yoga (the yoga of skilful and mindful action), as well as with ideas about the law of karma and intentions behind our actions: positive, negative or neutral.

Because of its links with the conscious mind and the world of thought, yoga – most famously the *Bhagavad Gita* – associates it with the intellect (*buddhi*, which at its highest level manifests wisdom) and makes connections with jnana yoga: the cultivation of discernment and high levels of intuitive knowledge. But beneath conscious activity there are unconscious influences affecting our aspirations and aims which motivate our will's energy. If we consider how different cultures, people and communities have different ideals and possessions they value, such as money or being compassionate to all beings, we see how this can influence their conscious actions and subconscious drives. It is, therefore, important to look at our values and other areas that affect us if we are to successfully proceed in spiritual development.

If used skilfully the will can serve as an important part of our development. My own creative background has taught me how the individual will can lead to different levels where the Creative Will takes over. For as long is it more purely predominant, this Creative Will, I find, always has less of a sense of self about it and can flow with its own constructive purpose and direction.

Practices such as one-pointed meditation are seen to strengthen the will. It is also through the will's use that we are able to focus our minds in periods of introspection, contemplation and meditation and shift our awareness to balanced states of mindfulness. The *Bhagavad Gita* says, "Let the man uplift the self by the self". In other words, use the individual will to awaken to wider states of being and understanding, including the higher Divine Consciousness and Its Creativity and harmonising influence – something which M. P. Pandit also reminds us of in his *Yoga in Savitri*:

> *The seeker has to learn to watch himself, impose his central will upon all his members and hold himself open in an act of surrender to the higher action.*

The will is particularly active in personal discipline – which encompasses patience and should not be confused with suppression or force – and can lead us to discovering and finally surrendering our individual will to deeper, more universal and less self-centred interests, and living more freely, openly and compassionately in the present. If developed and used in a skilful way, the will can help us to change restrictive patterns in our lives.

This may sound like a restriction on our freedom, but it actually gives us more flexibility and choice, whereas an undisciplined mind and life will have little direction. Instead of being overwhelmed by emotional upsets, restricted by a limited mind-set or unhealthy patterns, we are able to influence how we respond to life and events in more resourceful ways. The world will then benefit more from our actions, because our actions will have a greater impact for good; for, "A spiritual life without discipline is impossible", says Henri Nouwen.

Other areas of development and states of mind and heart are important, such as contemplation and being in harmony with life, but without a level of skilful mastery over ourselves we may find that we keep falling back into old ways of thinking and behaving. Life is not always about 'going with the flow'! Yet the will's development needs aspects of flexibility and spontaneity to guard against becoming rigid and narrowly focused. As Jung reminded us, "there are higher things than the ego's will, and to these one must bow".

Obviously spirituality is not always about being physically active. Traditionally there have always been stopping places where a traveller takes stock and looks back. Moments of reflection, rest and healing are essential, particularly if we have recently been through or come to terms with a stressful period in our spiritual journey.

There are also occasions when the will's energy deserts us. There are often good reasons why this happens. We may find that it is being blocked or suppressed because of fears that need acknowledging, or because we have been going in a direction that feels contrary to our nature or natural abilities. It can also be a way for different parts of ourselves to attract our attention in order to lead us to deeper understanding. It might even be that we have pushed ourselves too hard and need time to regenerate. If this is so, we could question why we have done this and not searched for a more balanced life. We need to ask what issues are behind the actions that have led us to be so harsh on ourselves.

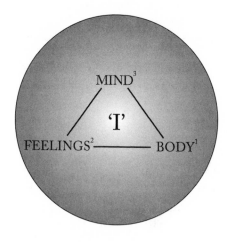

The circle represents the subconscious and unconscious mind that lies beneath the conscious levels of 'I', body (including the physical senses), feelings and mind (perceptual, thinking and reasoning abilities).

The numbers 1 to 3 show the order of natural development.

FIGURE 1:
Average Field of Awareness

Embracing wholeness

The difference between having a healthy or an unhealthy understanding of who we are and of our relationship with life and people, lies in being open to meaningful interaction with everyday experience rather than being shutdown in separation, unwholeness and unrealistic projections that isolate us from greater fields of being.

In our evolvement from our mother's womb, it is recognised that we move from body consciousness, to emotional consciousness and to mental consciousness (numbers 1 to 3 in *figure 1*), forming a triangle that creates individual consciousness and the connections between internal and external awareness. Over the last thirty years writers on spirituality have come to see the importance of developing a strong, healthy, mature and grounded individual sense of self that embraces everyday life in unafflicted ways, before aiming for transcendent states of awareness. The phrase, "You have to become someone before you become no one", comes to mind.

Problems can arise from any area: from the body, the mind, feelings or emotions. But we could spend a lifetime trying to therapeutically fix everything that has happened in our lives before considering wider realms of development and, if we are not careful, we can become side-tracked and stuck at a basic stage of growth that stops us from realising different ways of engaging with life. An example of this is when old dysfunctional patterns are used to hide in as a way of avoiding wider possibilities of development.

Here we need to be careful of over-identifying with and holding onto our wounds and limiting beliefs, instead of letting go and opening up to new experience and growth. Sometimes it feels safer to have the hurt that gives us a familiar sense of ourselves than exploring new ground. Rather like Picasso, who when asked what made a good painting, replied, "Knowing when to stop", we have to be aware of when to move on in our development.

Yet moving forward can, unfortunately, also present us with problems, which is why development is an ongoing process that may require different things at different times, such as strong social communities to support us, friends to share our troubles, rational stimulation that might help us to see life from wider perspectives, deep reflection about ourselves, or practical help with our spiritual practices: meditation, methods of prayer, guided reading, performing responsible actions in the world and finding unity with others.

If we embrace the whole – including higher qualities of mind, intuition, wisdom, reasoning, reflective thinking, compassion and the true Self – in order to untangle ourselves from unconscious fears and conditioned patterns of action and reaction, from grasping for pleasure or rejecting things when they do not fit our current understanding, we will arrive at a more centred and nourishing place. In the midst of unfamiliarity we can tap into the power of authentic being instead of obscuring it, and face and work through denied levels, difficult stages, and find ways of opening up to ourselves and others – allowing people in to touch our lives and to give help freely when others may need it.

There will of course be times when we feel impelled to revisit old wounds, to work more on our will, reassess our needs and become aware of reoccurring cycles and patterns. All this is a natural part of the development process, because in it there is an ongoing need to re-evaluate the past and the present from new perspectives that have been achieved.

The triple self

Figure 1, depicting the average field of awareness, shows how the body with its physical senses is connected with the mind (perceptions, memory and intellect), feelings, moods and emotions (the emotions being heightened and more intense feelings, whereas moods, such as peacefulness, are less intense and longer lasting).

All can be observed interrelating and affecting one another. For instance, when we experience something through our physical senses, the mind will invariably draw upon past memory and experience and decide whether it is pleasant or desirable, or not. Our emotions will often then respond according to our previous encounter and knowledge. However, it should be mentioned there are some emotions that are universally innate, such as surprise, joy, distress, fear and disgust, which do not necessarily rely on prior experience. The universal emotional expressions of babies confirm this. On the other hand, feelings of romantic love, envy, pride and embarrassment rely on high cognitive processes which babies have not developed.

We can also see how the emotions affect our mind when an overwhelming feeling or emotion comes to the surface. I am sure we can all recall moments when our common-sense has gone out of the window when we have fallen in love or had a crush on someone or lost our tempers. The mind, feelings and emotions also affect the body, as seen in times of stress and emotional conflict. Additionally, the body also has an affect on other areas. For instance, when we smile it produces endorphins in the brain that are involved in states of euphoria.

There can be a danger in seeing some of these levels as less important than others, or simplistically jumping on one as an explanation for any imbalance. The body has especially been looked down on in some traditions and the mind can be seized upon as an explanation for problems that may have physical origins. Sometimes mental growth is ignored in favour of a return to the emotional self. Although work on the emotions is important, but just as the mind can unhealthily suppress emotional maturity, so too can the emotions be used to avoid healthy mental growth.

The mind and emotions were once seen as two conflicting poles that could not be balanced and would always interfere with the development of each other. But this view no longer fits with contemporary understanding.

Recognising our many selves and overcoming conditioning

Much of what we may identify as being who we are is really a product of past actions, influences and self-imposed limitations. Where individual and spiritual growth can come together is in looking at how these affect us, our beliefs about ourselves and others, and discovering ways of untangling ourselves from unhealthy patterns.

I have already mentioned how we will define ourselves as being this or that type of person, as extrovert, introvert, shy, artistic and so on. The reality is that we have so many different qualities and personalities we draw upon and slip in and out of, they could fill an entire football stadium. Similar to Lewis Carol's Alice, we might catch ourselves wondering if we are the same person that got up this morning!

Contemporary psychology terms these aspects of ourselves as 'subpersonalities' and tells us that we need to be aware of them in order to learn about ourselves, and how to balance and integrate them into a synthesised whole. Various activities for doing this can include seeing which ones are major players and giving them names – sometimes humorous ones, which helps to make awareness of ourselves an enjoyable growing process – such as the carer, the artist, the critic, the athlete, the mystic and so on.

We will notice that they connect with different areas of our life and qualities of our nature, as seen in the suggested names and can, until healthily integrated, be a help or hindrance to living a productive spiritual life. Yet even the most creative is only a facet of the whole of who we are and will cause problems if we over-identify with it.

The idea of there being different qualities or states that we slip in and out of can be traced back to Buddhist notions connected with the Wheel of Life. It is often depicted in paintings of Mara (a demon-like figure personifying death) holding a large circle divided into sections, showing different domains, such as the realm of the hungry ghosts, fighting demons, heavenly beings and the animal kingdom. On the one hand, each section of the Wheel can be seen as depicting different worlds that people can be born into; on the other, they can be interpreted as psychological states that we encounter numerous times a day.

In Hindu philosophy there is the belief in the three *gunas* (explained in detail in the *Our Limitless Inheritance* chapter), which are seen to be active in different states that influence us in an infinite number of ways. We may think we are the same person all the time. But if we become aware of our everyday selves, we may notice that one minute we are behaving like a Buddha or a heavenly being, the next, like a fighting demon or a hungry desirous ghost.

Harmonisation

The approach of a healthy holistic and integral path is to honour and respect all aspects of our nature. There may be times when we discover we are in disharmony and find it difficult to accept conflicting parts. We might even impose an ideal image of how we think we should be and become disheartened when we don't live up to this.

While running a workshop on exploring sub-personalities with some students, one woman suddenly spoke up saying, "That can't be right, I have qualities that are the complete opposite of others!" This was a breakthrough for the student and an important step in the exercise to help people recognise, own, understand and balance the many and sometimes opposing parts of their life – including those that are not always easy to accept.

The One that unites and creates

Numerous Western psychologists have taken an interest in Eastern wisdom and its understanding of the individual 'I', how we process physical experience and how these are continuously changing. Yet this does not imply that individuality and the world of matter do not exist or can have a wholesome function to perform. Ultimately our individual natures and the physical universe are all unique facets of One Supreme Reality manifesting in Creation and need to be healthily included in spiritual growth.

Some teachings have encouraged the idea of there being a separation between nature and spirituality, or have promoted ideas about the meaninglessness of life. In opposition to these, wholism is about seeking an integration of our being with nature and being more life affirming. Now, more than ever, we need to include and cherish the Earth and all its inhabitants, instead of denying and/or abusing our planet and not caring about our global brothers and sisters. For teachers such as Sri Aurobindo, spirituality is about being one with all nature and all beings. Indeed, in our deepest depth we are one with all creatures and the Divine.

Some contemporary Christian teachers, such as Matthew Fox, have encouraged seekers to recognise their interconnected relationship with all, and to revere and celebrate this unique interaction. The sacredness and beauty of nature are after all, expressions of God's Creative, eternal Goodness. For Christians it may be seen as the Word or the presence of the Cosmic Christ/immanent God Consciousness in all things that unites all humanity. It is the Self of all: the One which each of us participates in and gives meaning and purpose to life. The medieval mystic Hildegarde of Bingen pointed out that, "The Word is living, being, spirit, all verdant greening, all creativity. This Word manifests itself in every creature".

In the influential work of Teilhard de Chardin, the two worlds of the universal Spirit and individuality are looked upon as inseparable:

> *Purity does not lie in separation from, but in a deeper penetration into the universe. It is to be found in the love of that unique boundless essence which penetrates the inmost depths of all things and there, from within those depths, deeper than the mortal zone where individuals and multitudes struggle, works upon and moulds them. Purity lies in a chaste contact with that which is 'the same in all'.*
>
> Pierre Teilhard de Chardin

Even in the midst of one of the darkest wars in history, Teilhard de Chardin was able to write and affirm, "There is a communion with God, and a communion with earth, and a communion with God through earth".

Although natural disasters demonstrate a destructive side to nature – just as our own creativity can have when it is manifested without responsibility and a spiritual purpose – it is because of our connections with nature that we find it so healing and often feel pulled to reflect upon its abundant beauty. No two humans or blades of grass are identical, yet all connect with an underlying unity. If meditated upon, the smallest plant or creature can lead us to realising deeper mysteries and how we are not separate from each other. Because of this connection, we have an individual and collective responsibility for humanity and the world, as we are all one family created in God with infinite creative potential, which we were given to use.

Spirituality is in many ways about being awake to this potential, and the abilities and possibilities that are available to us in every moment, which can lead us to being spontaneously creative and skilfully participating in life as it unfolds. For within everyone there is the Creative Divine Impulse, and when we create, we are taking part in and celebrating the Creativity that exists within the universe – we become co-Creators.

This active form of spirituality is intrinsically bound up with wholeness and compassion. We should not confuse it with egotistical ideas of creativity, but realise that it is to do with what can naturally flow from us as a result of our interrelation with all. It connects us to the dance of Creation in the quest for cosmic harmony and balance. Through this we find a deeper sense of the sacred in all. For as the social and spiritual activist Vimala Thakar reminds us, "As soon as there is awareness of wholeness, every moment becomes sacred, every moment is sacred".

This all links with ideas on Creation Spirituality, which Matthew Fox has done much to bring our attention to in recent years. Its roots are found not only in the Christian mystical tradition, but also in Tantric yoga, connected with various chakras and with Shakti (the Creative Divine Mother energy), and with aspects of Sufi, Buddhist, Taoist, ancient Celtic, African, Australian Aboriginal, Native American Indian and Hasidic Jewish spirituality. It is seen as being as old as Creation itself, because of its connections with the Creative Force and Mind that has pervaded the universe since its birth.

3

Transformations in Development

SWAMI DHARMANANDA

What do the seasons mean to you? Spring, for instance, we may see as a time of hope, subsidence of storms, spring cleaning and preparation of the ground for sowing new seeds. Each season has its trademark, its own particular meaning and purpose for the continuity and the creativity of nature. We too may go through various seasons of sadness and joy. Let us look at these times, feelings, thoughts and qualities within us and use them for learning more about life in all dimensions. By doing so we can become more spiritually aware of the different forces within us and start to change our overall levels of being.

We all go through various light and dark periods in our development. This is to be expected as we grow out of old patterns of thinking and behaviour, and life wakes us up to a greater truth and reality. For within the darkness of winter there dwells the light of spring and growth.

Development is about bringing together all our experiences of life and being at one with them. After winter look to new vision, new light, new life. Sow and you shall reap the rewards of spiritual growth, happiness and enlightenment.

An evolving cycle of change

We may experience many different cycles of change. Sometimes we can become complacent and hibernate for periods in our development, and maybe gather a little dust around our spiritual light. But even if the mirror of our soul has become a bit murky, we now might be thinking that it is time to cast off the wraps, to dust ourselves down and to get polishing, so that we can open up to the Sun in our life and start working towards reflecting a shining Divine Light and mirror the

Supreme Spirit more clearly.

One important thing we can do for nourishment is to study the spiritual texts. If we study the *Patanjali Sutra*, particularly the *yamas* (external ethical virtues) and *niyamas* (cultivation of inner virtues) – outlined by Santoshan in the *Steps to Authentic Being* chapter – we will learn about the essentials for living a spiritual life. The *yamas* and *niyamas* outline a way of action, a way of spiritual cleansing and remind us about higher levels of being and consciousness.

The *Bhagavad Gita* also shows various roads that can be taken which lead to ultimate union with God and all that is within and around us. The ethics of yoga spirituality show a way of life, a way of knowing ourselves, of relating to others and realising a profound inner peace which helps us through the obstacles and upheavals of life.

In order to uphold the basic precepts of yoga, we need to expand our awareness and observe life and ourselves reflectively, and learn about our strengths and weaknesses – using our strengths to transform the appearance of any inhibiting qualities within us.

The path to spiritual awareness may not always be easy, but have faith and God will be your guide, help and strength. Use the power of prayer and you will find that God will be even closer than you may realise.

Sowing the seeds of growth

In our lives we sow many seeds; some seeds mature and some wither. Some seeds grow into delicate flowers, small bushes and mighty trees. We may sow seeds that hinder and stifle the growth of the plants of beauty, and those that give comfort, shelter and nourishment – to both ourselves and others. And so we need to look at our garden of life, and to weed out carefully the seeds of discontent, envy, hatred, anger, jealousy and others that inhibit our growth. We then need to nourish the plants of light and love, and sow the seeds of acceptance, contentment, and others that bring forth their fragrance, comfort and nourishment and help to others. Through this we may look at our garden and see the growth that has taken place, which will then produce seeds for further potential, evolvement and fulfilment. The student who embraces all life as a part of the growing process, will always move forward in his or her evolvement.

Nurturing the good

To me the following quotation is a summary of yoga:

> *Chant the name and praise of the Lord, and sing His glory.*
> *Meditate on His divine attributes,*
> *constantly remember Him and His Presence.*
> *Serve and worship the Lord of Love.*
> *Bow down to Him; know Him as the true friend,*
> *surrender yourself unto Him.*
> *The whole universe may be compared to a large tree.*
> *All beings may be said to be its leaves and branches.*
> *Hari, God, is the root of the tree.*
> *When the Lord is worshipped all beings rejoice.*
> SRIMAD BHAGAVATAM

Whichever path we have chosen, whatever religion or our nationality, 'yoga is for all'. It is the path of union of our individual self with the transcendent and universal Self: the recognition of our true spiritual being – That which is a part of God. For we were all made in the likeness of the Creator.

When the tree casts its seeds then those seeds grow into the likeness of the tree. But just as these seeds need to be nourished, we must also cultivate the Divine Seed within us. Although all practices of yoga can help us to do this, we will often need to rely on more than one method. The *Hatha Yoga Pradipika* states that the physical postures are, "only for the attainment of Raja Yoga", reminding us that we must go beyond, as well as include, the physical to understand the Divine and Its deepest implications.

The *yamas* and *niyamas* are a guide to conduct that will help us along the path to Self-realisation. *Pranayama* exercises help us to understand the energies both within ourselves and universally. They help us to move toward the union of the material, psychic and spiritual planes of existence. Meditation practices supplement this by bringing us closer to Divine knowledge and Divine realisation.

When we look at the mistakes we have made in our lives, the anguish or hurt we may have caused others, or things we have done which we are not proud of, we can sometimes understandably find it hard to recognise our spiritual nature. But through prayer and meditation we can come to the sanctuary of the Divine and find forgiveness. "The real way of profiting by the humiliation of one's own faults is to face them", Fenelon reminds us.

We must learn to forgive and love ourselves – warts and all – before we can transfer our forgiveness, love and compassion to others. We should never despair, but endeavour to keep evolving and growing. Learn to be kind to yourself and to cultivate the healing power of self-acceptance; for we cannot change anything until we know how to accept it. Realise you are more than the appearance of any negatives, and being aware of and working with and through them is the core of practical development. Go to the roots of the tree and find nourishment there. This is yoga and spiritual growth in action. Realise what is meant by the mantra *So-ham* (I am That); that ultimately you are a pure spark of the Divine.

For many years the *Srimad Bhagavatam* has been an inspiration and comfort to me. The love of the Divine and the teachings of Krishna are shown so strongly. I therefore give thanks to the Divine souls who passed on these words and teachings: "The highest duty of life is to take delight in the Word of God and to meditate constantly upon Him as the embodiment of all Truth." For if God is in all things, and all things are in God, then the Divine is forever revealing Itself in the world and through the teachings and lives of those who have been touched by Its creative influence.

Transforming ourselves in the Light of the true Self

Changes are inevitable if we are to continue to grow in the knowledge and application of yoga. Remember yoga is about life, and the practices are for growth and for expanding our spiritual awareness. I would be failing in the work my Guru Paramahansa Satyananda gave me to carry out if I did not endeavour to convey this and, indeed, aim to live by it. My teacher Sri Trivadi Ramachandra also wanted me to encourage all students I came into contact with, to convey the true essence of the practices – the essence that is portrayed in the teachings of the *Vedas*, *Upanishads*, *Gita*, *Great Epics*, *Tantras* and many spiritual writings.

Within these teachings it reminds us that we are pure Spirit here and now. They advocate practices that help us to awaken to the infinite qualities of the Spirit within and reveal Its true radiance. The mantra *So-ham* can help us do this by reminding us of the ever-present Divine. It is within everyone's capabilities to be able to chant this mantra, or to contemplate it silently on the in and out flow of breath (*'So'* on the in-breath and *'ham'* on the out-breath).

By daily chanting the *Gayatri*, it can help to remove obstacles and bring us closer to that Great Union, the Ultimate Yoking/Integration of our being with the true Self – realising That which we know as God, the Divine Light. The *Gayatri* (*Om bhur bhuvah swah, tat savitur varenyam; bhargo devasya dhimahi, dhiyo yo nah prachodayat*) is one of the oldest mantras in the *Rig Veda* and can roughly be translated as, 'Oh Creator of the universe we meditate on Thy supreme splendour; may Thy radiant Light illuminate our intellect and guide us in the right direction'. Through meditation, mantra and profound and deep levels of prayer we can become instruments of God's compassion, forgiveness, light, joy, peace and love.

We need to offer ourselves in service and share the truth and wisdom of yoga in all areas of our lives and in all that we do:

Whatever actions I may perform
Impelled by the forces of Nature
By body, word, mind, senses, intellect, Soul
I offer to the feet of the Divine Lord.
TRADITIONAL PRAYER

Knowing ourselves and manifesting the Divine in everyday life

If we look at what has occurred over the centuries and learn from the mistakes that humankind has made, we may one day be able to achieve a true peace that everyone can benefit from. Humankind needs to use its scientific and spiritual discoveries to help and benefit humanity and the world. Not for the purpose of destruction, but for progress, growth and spiritual advancement in order to create a better place to live and achieve a closer bond with each other and nature.

We all need to work harder to understand our relationship

	POSITIVE	NEGATIVE
TO ONESELF	*Self-knowledge, self-acceptance and realising positive potential*	*Lack of healthy awareness, and an inability to change and express oneself wholesomely*
TO LIFE	*Finding fulfilment, meaning and purpose*	*Trivial preoccupations that lack positive direction*
TO NATURE	*Caring for and living in harmony with it*	*Harming and selfishly destroying its natural balance*
TO OTHERS	*Manifesting compassion, understanding and respect*	*Stereotyping and generalising about people*
TO PROBLEMS	*A time for learning and growing*	*Unable to see alternative perspectives and accept that nothing stays the same*
TO SPIRITUALITY	*Integrating all parts, continuously evolving and awakening to the sacred in all*	*Beliefs that separate us from one another and our responsibility for the Earth*

FIGURE 2: *Positive and Negative Approaches.*

with God, the created universe, life and our authentic spiritual Self. Through the Union/Yoga of our physical, emotional, intellectual and spiritual being we can bring about harmony within and so manifest a unity that reaches out to include others. Only through knowing ourselves can we begin to know God. The work is always ongoing, a constant awareness and consciousness of the living presence of God that works and expresses Its sacdredness through all. Let us start a new era with the determination to look at ourselves, and overcome the everyday problems that disharmoniously separate us from one another. Let us grow in love, compassion and peace, and start a new beginning with the intention of spreading our unitive and creative abilities and attributes in order to achieve a greater spiritual awareness in the world.

Figure 2 was influenced by a diagram in A. S. Dalal's *Looking from Within* and is a brief summary of some attitudes to bear in mind.

Readers will no doubt think of others that could be added.

Balancing the complete self

When we compare the wisdom and science of the ancient cultures we find that they have much in common. The rishis, the priests, the physicians, the wise men and women in these cultures considered the body, mind and Spirit needed to work in harmony to be in a balanced state – that the intrinsic inner energies needed to be used and directed correctly.

They recognised the links between movement, breath and sound, and how these can affect various physical organs and psychic energy centres within us. They discovered that by directing *prana* (or *chi*) energies – both physically and mentally – they can bring about a balance needed for an overall well-being of the physical, mental and spiritual levels of ourselves. These cultures and teachings contributed to the knowledge and practices that are still being used today – truth never dies it seems – to help humankind. So when we receive and practise these ancient teachings, we must surely treasure them.

Integrating the teachings

May my word be one with my thought,
and my thought be one with my word, O Lord of Love.
Let me realise you in my consciousness.
May I realise the truth of the scriptures
and translate it into my daily life.
AITAREYA UPANISHAD

Let us encourage ourselves and others to band together in our work and radiate out like the spokes of a wheel. The wheel can be seen to contain the essence of yoga, the spiritual centre of the Self, which we are all a part of. Yoga in its truest form is ultimately a way of life. We may practise *asanas*, *pranayama*, mindfulness and meditation, but unless we carry the formula of the *yamas* and *niyamas* into our daily lives, the essence fades. Without the *yamas* and *niyamas* we will not be able to achieve a true spiritual awareness that looks deeply into life.

The practices are there to help us tap into inner knowledge of the true Self and our interactive relationship with all. They give us strength during adversity, and courage to overcome the obstacles that confront and often appear to bind or restrict us.

The teachings of yoga and those in various wisdom traditions are there to guide us on our way and remind that the spiritual life is forever in the 'here and now'. We may have plans for the future, but we can only act on those plans according to the present moment.

By working on our unfoldment, embodying the teachings, opening our hearts, being mindful and aware of each passing phase or season of life, and through practising God Consciousness, we can rise above entanglements, heal our mental and emotional wounds, and help and inspire others in much freer, compassionate and creative ways.

4
Love is Only Part of it

SANTOSHAN

Since writing the last book with Glyn Edwards I have given talks on the model briefly outlined in its introduction (adaptation below) and have received questions from students and readers interested in learning more about the way various levels tie-up with one another, how they can be unpacked and expanded further and linked with different wisdom traditions. The point made in the book with Glyn about every level intertwining and there being no absolute boundary between them – as there are rainbows within rainbows of awareness within each, which will affect one another in various ways – still applies. As an example of this, modern psychology has discovered that rational thinking cannot happen without the interaction of the emotions.

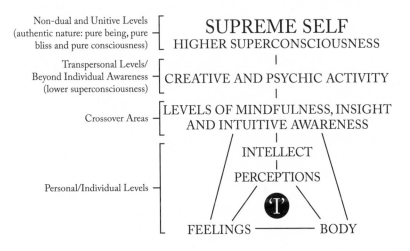

FIGURE 3: *Interconnected Paths and Levels of Awareness.*

I make no apologies for the model being a multidimensional one that draws on hierarchical language and structure; though ultimately there is no above, below or behind in the essential oneness of our universal nature. But it gives us a symbolic and metaphorical handle to discuss aspects of ourselves that fall into different categories of Ultimate Being and relative existence. All language can be seen as metaphor anyway, and metaphor and symbolism are the languages of the psyche.

The alternative is to reduce everything to a single realm, which fails to acknowledge what makes us human, i.e. our ability to rise above our materialistic nature, use our communication and reasoning skills, as well as reflect and have a spiritual dimension to life.

Modern reductionist thinking will not consider these as different levels and invariably seeks to shrink all aspects of consciousness, emotional and spiritual life to the realms of such things as biology and behavioural science – treating inner spiritual experiences as having no ultimate reality because of their subjective nature.

People seeking a post-modern 'no truths' approach tell us that, "The only thing we can be absolutely sure of, is there is nothing we can be absolutely sure of". As this idea seeks to be an absolute itself, it logically follows that it also cannot be relied upon as a statement of truth and is, therefore, a nonsensical statement.

Interestingly, some holistic and surprisingly transpersonal and spiritual groups have knowingly or unknowingly been influenced by such views and are occasionally suspicious of any model with the hint of a graded approach and belief in the reality of a higher life. Their focus, although including elements of transcendence, is often primarily in the relative area of discovering one's *own truth* – even though one would often be expected to take on the group's truth about development – and the ongoing process of becoming: becoming more balanced, well-rounded, etc. Important as this area of development is, and it should not be left out, as there are truths that only relate to us that we need to explore, it supplies us with only a partial understanding and tells us little about ultimate levels of being. The following extract from E. F. Schumacher best selling *Small is Beautiful* takes a more pragmatic stand:

... the notion of an hierarchical order is an indispensable instrument of understanding. Without the recognition of 'levels of Being' or 'Grades of Significance' we cannot make the world intelligible to ourselves nor have we the slightest possibility to define our own position, the position of man in the scheme of the universe.

Practical evolvement

In the process of spiritual development we not only have to be aware of the physical and everyday psychological influences in our lives, and recognise any agenda that may lie behind our perspectives on life, but also we have to grow beyond them.

Initially we will have to accept and explore the experiences that have led us to where we are now, as these are our stories, our life histories and narratives which we use to justify our temperament and views. Eventually we will discover they are only partial realities which do not supply us with a complete or very clear picture. Nonetheless, we will not be able to travel far unless we assess the roads that have brought us to this moment and understand something about the way we work – physically, emotionally and mentally – and how to move forward and become more spiritually whole and creative.

Effective meditative awareness practices, or work with a skilled therapist, will look behind our stories and at areas of over-identification, attachment, fear, delusion, misconceptions, unnecessary suffering, self-imposed limitations and how to be free of them.

The body and paths of action

There are obviously many paths to consider when it comes to the body, such as hatha yoga and tai chi that can help us become aware of our physical and spiritual selves. Yet though the body's senses are the prime gateways to exterior experience, our perceptions are rarely pure, as they are highly influenced by our stored knowledge, assumptions, memories and past experience.

It is through awareness of our senses and perceptions that we become more skilfully conscious of life and how we relate to it. This helps us not only to open up, but also to become more responsible for our actions and empathic with other's needs and suffering; making us more caring, kind, compassionate, spiritually aware and mature human beings. In essence, this is the practice of karma yoga (Buddhist might think more in terms of skilful actions and ethical obligations) in its broadest and most practical sense. The parable of the good Samaritan demonstrates how compassionate actions are more important than beliefs and rituals and is something we should not forget.

Awareness of our physical selves is also important for helping us become sensitive to any stress that is affecting the body and the immune system, or physical problems affecting other states of being. For if our bodies are suffering and causing us pain, then our emotional and mental well-being will invariably be affected.

Tension held in the body can be connected with past or present trauma and released through body-work – such as breath awareness, dance or simply learning how to relax – by bringing awareness to any tension, pain or discomfort and discovering what wounds may lie beneath and how to let go of them. Mindfulness meditation and positive visualisation practices are invaluable for seeing what is going on within us and affirming our more healthy selves, and are medically known to help boost the immune system, calm the mind, body and emotions and help awaken us to fresher fields of growth.

Breathing exercises are particularly good for bringing attention to the present moment and helping us surrender to an eternal unconditioned 'now'. They are also a bridge to the emotional body, as the rhythm of our breathing automatically alters as our emotions change and we can bring about peaceful states through focusing on the breath, which affect the way we respond to life within and around us.

Practising the path of love

As well as being an area for individual emotional growth, the feeling part of ourselves links with practices of compassion and bhakti yoga – the yoga of unconditional devotion and surrender to God, and seeing and honouring the Divine in all things and people. When bhakti yoga is practised at its highest it leads to loving and compassionate acts of kindness in all areas of life.

'But what does unconditional love mean?', a friend recently asked. Firstly, we should not confuse it with sexual attraction. Neither is it a love that confines itself to only those closest to us or to a select few that we admire. The word 'agape' is used by Christians to distinguish it from these things. If we consider the work of Mother Teresa of Calcutta we will have some understanding of its implications. A passage from the Old Testament, "I have heard you calling me in the night; if you lead me I will hold your people in my heart", comes to mind.

But to truly open our hearts, the psychological self invariably needs working on in order to overcome petty prejudices and stereotypes that stop us from connecting with others and acting in a kind, caring and friendly way. The reflective mind also needs to be incorporated to help us be realistic about ourselves, our actions and reactions, and understand something about the way we respond to people in all walks of life. This requires being gentle on ourselves, as there are often good reasons why we are the way we are and our spiritual potential is unable to manifest in some situations. We, therefore, need to generate love, compassion and friendliness towards ourselves. In fact we cannot have love for others unless we know how to do this – our well will be empty.

We cannot force ourselves to develop these gifts. For they must arise naturally within our hearts as a response to our interconnectedness with all and the sharing in others' pains and joys, and through the use of other spiritual qualities, such as understanding and non-judgment. "Compassion is a spontaneous movement of wholeness", Vimala Thakar reminds us, and happens automatically when this wholeness is realised and lived. Similarly, Matthew Fox points out, compassion is, "the working out of our connectedness; it is the praxis of interconnectedness".

Work towards this understanding and compassionate way of being can be cultivated by finding ways to touch life more deeply through creativity, meditation, widening our understanding, affirmations, profound states of contemplative prayer, therapeutic work and social responsibility. The psychologist John Welwood made the following observation in his *Journey of the Heart*:

> *Whenever our heart opens to another person, we experience a moment of unconditional love. People commonly imagine that unconditional love is a high or distant ideal, one that is difficult,*

if not impossible, to realise. Yet though it may be hard to put into every day practice, its nature is quite simple and ordinary: opening and responding to another person's being without reservation.

We must realise that our true nature unites us with everything in the universe. To manifest and reflect this intrinsic part of ourselves we need to overcome the boundaries that separate us. But compassion can sometimes mean saying 'No' to help someone become more self-reliant, or honour our own selves if people are abusing our good nature – wisdom plays its role here and always needs to accompany spiritual practices.

The path of love, in its truest sense, connects with both the body and the mind; for it requires knowledge and understanding of our true Self and its implications (the path of jnana yoga), which naturally leads to the practice of unconditionally giving one's self and altruistic actions in the world (the path of karma yoga practised in an ethical way). We see from this how bhakti, karma and jnana yoga automatically overlap if practised at their highest level.

The unfolding work

The initial stages of working on ourselves are about acknowledgment. If a negative rises to the surface, we must acknowledge any hurt, fear, anger or insecurities, and realise it is an opportunity for growth, understanding and transformation. If we are sincere and let things in, give them some room and own them without judgment, instead of ignoring or suppressing them, we can begin the healing process.

Instead of thinking there is something wrong when we feel cut-off, needy or agitated, and placing conditions on how we image we or things should be, we accept life and ourselves in all dimensions.

A sense of spaciousness can be experienced as we release any tension or negatives and become aware of richer fields of existence. We may at first feel like avoiding a part of our life because it feels too painful to embrace, or fight against opening ourselves, as it means entering unfamiliar territory. We might even attempt justifying our negatives, or make light of things that have happened to us as a way of not being in touch with our feelings, thoughts and concerns. But we will discover that connecting fully with ourselves – meaning more than just the shadow side of our personality – leads to a fullness and wholeness where we are no longer separated from the experience of truly living. I like the way A. H. Almass described this in his *Spacecruiser Inquiry*:

> *When the dynamism of our Being unfolds our experience in its dark and negative possibilities, we find ourselves trapped in repeating patterns and closed loops ...*
>
> *The situation is not hopeless, however, and we all know this some place in our hearts. We know – perhaps vaguely, perhaps incompletely – that the human spirit possesses the possibility of enlarging its experience, of opening up its richness.*

Although negatives obscure our true nature, in the Tantric tradition nothing is denied, suppressed or abandoned, but is included in order to bring about a total transformation of every facet of our being. This is not achieved through force. Negatives are surrendered to and realised that they do not exist as they appear. The path to growth lies in working through our inhibiting conceptions and emotions, as well as in finding and actualising the hidden creative potential underlying the issues that cause problems in our development.

Interestingly, two of the three *gunas* (qualities) that are mentioned in yoga – *rajas* (activities and passions) and *tamas* (dullness, inertia and ignorance) – are seen as energies behind emotions such as aggression and depression. Yet the third *guna*, *sattva* (purity), can awaken us to harmonious living.

By freshly evaluating restrictive emotions, feelings or thoughts, without involvement in any inhibiting stories we may give to them, we open up to ourselves and allow our troublesome areas room to truly communicate with us. In this process, we find that we are able to be authentic and feel a sense of release as we let old restrictive patterns go and allow a deep healing to take place. We may at first feel raw and exposed. But once we recognise inhibiting parts and realise them for what they are, we begin to see them as areas that can be changed and grown out of.

By exploring previously denied realms, we access our inner resources and unfold our own knowledge and wisdom about life and growth into true Selfhood. When we open up without attachment or judgment, we discover that beneath all our highs and lows there lies a deeper unconditional quality of aliveness, pure presence, peace and freedom – what Mahayana Buddhists understand as our inherent original nature and Hindu yogis consider as the true essence of the Self.

This essential level transcends restrictive patterns and is a realm of non-conceptual awareness, which has the ability to embrace, own, transform and harmonise all parts. We cannot force this to happen, but we can start putting things in place that lead to a spontaneous awakening to it and a freedom from the things that bind us.

The way of the mind or the way of no mind?

The starting place for mental spiritual growth is to ask the age old questions, 'Who am I?', 'Why am I here?', 'What do I need to do to change my overall understanding of myself and life?' and realise that although we have individual bodies, minds and feelings, they are only parts and expressions of a much greater reality. Reflections such as these help us to assess where we are now, how to move forward and awaken to transforming insights. For in truth, we are sparks of the Divine, interconnected with pure levels of creativity and consciousness.

Around the 5th century BCE there must have been something in the air for there to be such a huge shift from mythical ways of relating to the world to deep reflective insights. This can be traced back to not only the ancient Greek philosophers, but to India and China, to people such as the Buddha and Confucius.

The Buddha himself must have had remarkable mental powers to put together a wide system of thought and developmental ideas and practices in such a cohesive way. Of course Buddhism is not merely about mental growth and the Zen saying about it being, "A transmission beyond all words and scripture", reminds us of this. But no Buddhist monasteries are without at least one prime text that is studied alongside introspective practices. Clearly, the Zen saying is warning us not to allow the intellect to get in the way of other forms of development. However, it does not follow that we should not read, discuss deep issues, cultivate our reasoning and reflective abilities and come to our own understanding about spirituality.

The saying also draws our attention to the idea of 'sudden enlightenment' – the spontaneousness of Zen satori experiences – and beliefs about there being no need for a gradual path of evolvement. A theological comparison might be to think in terms of the Divine being 'here now', or the true Self being immanently present and all that has to be done is to realise this. However, we should be careful about abandoning ideas of evolvement, as the ego can play wonderful tricks on us when its regular life is threatened.

For the Zen practitioner, a satori/enlightenment experience might only happen after years of harsh training and may not always bring about a complete transformation. Buddhist writer Douglas M. Burns pointed out in his book *Nirvana, Nihilism and Satori* that while much concern is given to freeing oneself from the restrictive elements of intellectual thought in Zen, there is little advice given on bringing about positive changes in one's feelings and emotions.

Language and the way of unknowing
Language is often the starting place for many to learn about development. Used creatively it becomes a powerful tool for manifesting harmony within ourselves and the world. It helps us to identify and express abstract feelings, thoughts and experiences. Without words we will have little understanding of life and spiritual matters. Yet we may have to change our dialogue and interpretations to a more healthy and positive outlook if things are not working.

A problem with language occurs when we use it too loosely and fail to properly communicate, or try to escape into a purely intellectual approach to development. We have to know how to use language differently when talking about abstract feelings, thoughts and developmental experiences; otherwise we may end up like the main character in the old *Close Encounters* movie who raves wildly about seeing things like a 'Whoosh!' to his wife and children, who think he has completely lost the plot at this point in the film.

We can look at our dialogue and see if it matches our feelings. Often there is a superficial rationalisation that stops us from truly connecting. If we are honest and do not consciously know what is going on and admit that we are unaware of deeper aspects, we can at least proceed truthfully from this stage.

In John Welwood's *Towards a Psychology of Awakening* he mentions how phrases such as, 'I feel stupid', need exploring, as they do not describe feelings at all. Such phrases are used for avoiding emotional connection and need to be separated from what is really happening; for behind them there are true feelings and experiences that can be touched.

Welwood draws on the teachings of Shunryu Suzuki about original and beginner's mind and writes about arriving at a place of 'not knowing', where we are no longer the experts with beliefs in few choices in the routes to take in our life. It takes humility and maturity to admit that we do not have all the answers. Yet with these two qualities we are always open to development. Suzuki himself, pithily reminds us about this: "In the beginner's mind there are many possibilities, but in the expert's there are few." Once again this may give the impression of the intellect having no role to play.

Starting from the point of not knowing we come to realise that our conceptions and projections are cutting us off from reality. Here we discover a greater expanse of awareness beyond the world of thought with its limiting reactions and a more genuine way forward. It is a principal path mystics of various traditions have explored in contemplative and meditative practices – a way of emptying ourselves, or perhaps better explained as 'quietening the mind and letting go', and awakening to non-conceptual consciousness in moments of deep stillness.

It can often be a momentary state – unless it has been firmly established as a more definite stage of evolvement – where both the mind and heart open and we embrace the whole of ourselves in a unifying experience that leads to a profound oneness with life and transforming depths of pure awareness. It is a place where all ills come to rest and we surrender to the 'nowness' and true reality of the moment. For this to arise naturally we have to be careful not to imprison the splendour by expecting it to happen in a certain way or be the same experience as some other time.

When we awaken to this expanded state of openness, pure being and presence, we discover that it encourages an inclusive wholeness which helps us to let go of our fears, pains, restrictive patterns and anxieties. Instead of letting life close us down because it does not match our expectations, or allowing our life-stories and concepts to cut us off from fresh experience, we open up to the natural flow of existence and allow it to take us where we need to go. Through this we discover a clearness of vision and unrestrictiveness of heart that awakens us to uninhibited life, compassion and a true understanding of how things really are.

This all corresponds with Buddhist views on mindfulness, emptiness and enlightenment – which draw on negative terminology for descriptions of Ultimate Reality – where we are truly awake and have blown out the fires of ignorance, anger and desires of how we want things to be. We can also see how it links with the insights of the seers of the ancient *Upanishads*, who spoke of the Divine as 'pure being and pure consciousness' – which encompasses unconditional openness and presence – and 'pure bliss': love, joy and compassion.

The gifts of imagination and higher reasoning

Imagination can be viewed as either a help or a hindrance to development. On the one hand, it can distract us from being open to the present, and cause anxiety and false hopes when we preoccupy ourselves with thoughts about things that may never happen, or come up with all kinds of reasons to justify our hurts and defend our negatives. On the other hand, it is the force behind creativity. If used beneficially – and mixed with elements of intuitive insight, reflection and receptiveness to any openings – it plays a key role in development, especially in visualisation and therapeutic practices, such as evoking pleasant thoughts, seeing oneself on a spiritual quest or in another's shoes. It can move us from being egocentric and ethnocentric, where we only care about people in a closed circle of interest, to becoming more worldcentric, where we include all people and the welfare of the Earth.

Imagination and being receptive to insights can also involve picturing alternative goals and beneficial outcomes to the direction of our life and reflections on how to approach situations differently. It can help us re-evaluate our relationship with the Divine and be more inclusive and all-embracing in our understanding of spirituality.

Making the mind flexible

In yoga, different types of intelligence have long been recognised, such as ordinary intelligence (*apara-vidya*) and higher abilities of reflection that lead to spiritual wisdom (*para-vidya*). On a basic level it is often a lack of insight and understanding (*avidya*) that causes confusion, problems in our unfoldment, prejudice and a lack of acceptance of difference in the world – a refusal to see wider possibilities and alternative perspectives that would break down reactive, unthought-through generalisations. The Mother (Mira Alfassa) had this to say about us working on this level of ourselves:

> *In its natural state the human mind is always limited in its vision, narrow in its understanding, rigid in its conceptions, and a constant effort is therefore needed to widen it, to make it more supple and profound. So it is very necessary to consider everything from as many points of view as possible.*

By expanding the mind we can embrace life and others more healthily. In the excellent book *Destructive Emotions*, narrated by Daniel Goleman, it mentions the Tibetan Buddhist equivalent of a PhD, which can take up to thirty years to complete. Monks are asked to put forward complex philosophical ideas while others are encouraged to find fault with them. This helps them to contemplate the complexities of life, free the mind from holding onto concepts, develop openness, flexibility of thought and acceptance of other's opinions. They learn to agree to disagree without feeling insecurely challenged by another's point of view. The practice helps to cultivate 'unafflicted intelligence', which is highly valued in the Tibetan tradition; it is used as an aid to spiritual growth and maturity.

The path of jnana yoga is also about developing and transcending the mind, and is a way of realising Ultimate Truths through knowledge, discernment and discriminating wisdom and insight – realising the intrinsic interconnected Self in the heart of all life. It is a path of elevated and illumined thought that leads to discovering our universal and Ultimate Spiritual Nature.

The early mystic seers of the *Upanishads* and the philosopher

Shankara were fundamentally jnana yogis. The saying *"neti, neti"* (not this, not this) from the *Brihadaranyaka Upanishad*, is a philosophical denial of all that is not a pure reflection of the Supreme Self.

Including and transcending the intellect

Everyone has alternative beliefs and experiences to our own. If we have problems with this, then we will never find harmony in life. Conflicts are signals to look inside ourselves and see what needs to be done to manifest real peace. When the whole person is developed, it helps us to become more responsible and wiser human beings. No matter how negative our past has been, we will arrive at a place that does not judge by appearances, but accepts life and people as they are – understanding that everyone is uniquely different with alternative viewpoints to our own.

Due to our individuality, no one's evolvement is the same. We can all have different needs at different stages and may find that what is helpful for one, might not be for another. It is because we all tread our own unique paths that we sometimes arrive at opposing views. Here we must be watchful of taking an 'I'm right and you're wrong' approach. Deepak Chopra tells us that, "Finding the truth is not a matter of making anyone wrong, but of seeing how every belief can be expanded".

Different descriptions do not imply that we have not discovered real truths. We are possibly approaching things from alternative standpoints. A poet, botanist and geologist would all describe a mountain range differently and yet all views would be valid for different reasons. We might even find ourselves including previously opposing perspectives as we expand our awareness. So we see that the search for spiritual growth is not about running away from the reflective, reasoning and enquiring mind, but putting it to good use, learning how to include and balance it with the intuitive mind, make it more flexible and unafflicted.

There is obviously a difference between material rationalism and spiritual understanding. Whereas the first seeks to reinforce the divisions between us and all other life, the latter is open to inspiration and knowledge beyond itself, and looks for ways to overcome any separation. In Joseph Vrinte's *The Quest for the Inner Man* he feels that it is not by becoming irrational that one awakens to more unitive levels of consciousness, but by passing through reason to super-reason. In Thomas Keating's *The Human Condition*, he points out that in the Christian tradition, using reason to overcome aggression and immaturity is part of the practice of virtue – although we should remember that it can sometimes suppress emotions that need letting in and working through. As always it is about finding a balance.

The integral philosopher Ken Wilber has made useful observations and mentions how some mistakenly see spiritual growth as a return to a romanticised early/pre-personal state of evolvement that excludes intellectual realms of development. Confusion has arisen, he feels, because both the *pre*-personal (early childhood) and *trans*-personal (beyond individual consciousness) levels lean towards a state of oneness where there is a thin veil between the self and the world around it. However, at the *pre*-personal level this happens because the individual self and intellect have not developed, whereas at the *trans*-personal level they have not only reached a state of maturity, but have also been transcended.

Spiritual growth in this case is not a regression to an idealised childhood – which does not mean that we lose our sense of play, wonder and awe – but is an evolving process which takes us through many landscapes that includes, transforms and transcends the body, emotions and mind, instead of denying them, and awakens us to richer realms of being, wisdom, joy and understanding.

A final word is to mention that as we open to new life, there can be periods of struggle as old associations are changed. We may even find others feel threatened by our search. But as Glyn Edwards reminds us, "Development needs to be a courageous adventure where we dare to take risks and explore all possibilities, otherwise it is in danger of becoming uneventful and lacking positive direction".

The remaining parts to *figure 3* are discussed in the *Where Everything Interconnects* chapter.

5

Three Pillars of Wisdom

SWAMI DHARMANANDA

*Signs from the Soul come silently,
as silently as the sun enters the darkened world.*
TIBETAN SAYING

In the first chapter I wrote briefly about the importance of faith and its potential to help us in development. There are of course other essentials that are of great worth, such as the power of silence, the cultivation of peacefulness, and transforming our hearts, minds and different levels of being through what yoga describes as the practice of purification. It is these three areas that I will write about in this chapter and highlight their many advantages and dispel some misconceptions about them. Let us then look at the first all-important area of silence and stillness.

The empowering voice of silence
We can experience silence as both an internal and external quietness or calmness. There are many sayings and quotations stemming from the ancient texts, branching-out to our time through wise men, writers, poets, philosophers and even through some of our culture's popular songs – *The Sound of Silence* by Simon and Garfunkel for instance, and yes in some ways it can be heard – which try to convey the depth and meaning of silence.

Some students think that silence is not talking for a while. Of course this can be the beginning of the practice. Some think that as they are at home by themselves, without talking or listening to another person they are practising silence. But I wonder if the radio or television is used to provide background noise to replace the sound of a companion's voice. If this is the case, it is not 'the practice of silence'.

We need to be looking for a stillness within, through which we can come to discover the deeper aspects of ourselves. External silence will help us to find this internal state, but we must also quieten our minds, thoughts, physical actions and emotions in order to invoke an inner stillness, so that we can arrive at a deeper level of interior silence and discovery.

In most traditions silence is considered to be a necessary factor for all kinds of meditation practices that are undertaken in order to awaken to an awareness of the authentic Self. We need to immerse ourselves into silence so that we can become conscious of an inner world which transcends all conceptual understanding, and aware of the presence and influence of deeper levels of stillness which can transform our overall being.

In daily life we are constantly aware of external movements and sounds around us. In our post-modern world we are often bombarded with external sounds and distractions. Students tell me how it is becoming more difficult to 'get away from it all'. Yet ultimately the practice of silence leads us back into life with more peace and stability; for the practice of silence, which can also be called the practice of stillness, can be performed in the midst of noise and activity. But we first have to find that quiet centre within and establish it firmly in order to manifest it in everyday life. Going on a silent retreat can be extremely beneficial in helping us find this quality of silence which transcends everyday hustle and bustle.

Within yoga there are various practices designed to help us move along this path, such as the practice of *ajapa japa* (using sound as an instrument for spiritual development) and the practice of *antar mouna* (*antar* means inner; *mouna* means silence), which is used to bring about an awareness of external sounds that then leads to an inner awareness, for the purpose of attaining a state of internalised silence; thus we use that which might prevent us from knowing, experiencing and manifesting silence as a vehicle for achieving inner stillness. We, therefore, practise *mouna* (silence), then *antar mouna* (inner silence), and use sound itself to lead us to a deep level of stillness and quietness of the mind and the body.

These practices take us from the external to the internal, enabling us to become aware of our inner environment, thoughts, emotions and reactions. We then gradually refine our awareness of silence and fully enter into and become one with it – we realise that we are in fact part of the silence and it is part of us. The following quotation is by Paul Brunton, who uses the word 'Overself' to describe our higher spiritual nature in a poetic passage about silence:

We do not hear the sun rise,
So, too, the greatest moment in a man's life comes quietly.
In the stillness alone is borne the knowledge of the Overself.

The cultivation of a peaceful mind and heart

Another essential, which links with silence, is the cultivation of peacefulness. St. John of the Cross tells us the following about keeping peace in our hearts:

Keep your heart in peace; let nothing in this world disturb it; all things have an end.

In all circumstances, however hard they may be, we should rejoice, rather than be cast down, that we may not lose the greatest good, the peace and tranquillity of our soul …

… To endure all things with an equable and peaceful mind, not only brings with it many blessings to the soul, but also enables us, in the midst of our difficulties, to have a clear judgment about them, and to minister the fitting remedy for them.

Sorrow, sadness and wars are things in which, in one way or another, we are all involved. We all must pray for peace, whether internally or externally.

However, universal peace can only come when we are all at peace with ourselves. The New Testament and yogic texts point the way to achieving this. Jesus was a living example, and his sacred teachings live on as inspiring words that many have found helpful in times of inner turmoil, or external strife and conflict. Patanjali's *Yoga Sutra* summarises the eightfold steps of yoga. The *Bhagavad Gita* mentions several paths for finding inner peace. The *Tantras* also outline various practices, which can help us to eliminate discord within. So we see there is a path for everyone. But we must put whatever path we choose into action and then learn how to adapt it to different situations.

It is always nourishing when teachings are reflected upon for their deeper meanings, but to be truly effective, we must apply the basic precepts we find in the great traditions. The teachings are living things which are there for us to live by. It may be an act of faith (*shraddha*) or devotion, or something else that affects us internally which leads us to questions about life and to an awareness of the *atman*, the true Self, the Divine Spark in all.

All these things can be looked upon as aspects of the spiritual path (the *dharma marga*). Without spiritual precepts it is impossible to find a lasting peace, or indeed the Peace that passes all understanding – described by many true teachers of spirituality in all the great wisdom traditions.

If we practise with God Consciousness and develop even a small atom of peace within, we are helping to spread it. For we can only give what we have. With God Consciousness our yoga practice is not selfish, as we have reached a stage of maturity where we have woken-up to the reality of all things being interconnected and saturated in their Divinity. When we have this understanding, we no longer see ourselves as separate from others, or from their joys and pains.

Even if we do not fully realise Ultimate levels of being in this life, we may have been responsible for helping others to attain freedom and find peace in their lives; this is, after all, part of the noble path of the *bodhissatva* vow in Mahayana Buddhism and the important spiritual practice of compassion.

Yet we must always question our motives. Are we seeking peace because we want to escape from the world, or because we are seeking to contribute to life in creative ways? Are we seeking a selfish or an openly compassionate self-less spirituality?

Our intentions and aims need to be about cultivating a communal spirit of love, peace and harmony with all. We must strive to support each other in our joys and sorrows, our achievements and our difficulties along the path, and to generate spiritual awareness, as well as receiving and giving (being open to others and sharing our spiritual gifts), as an ongoing process that leads us to true peace and a loving unity with others:

Pray for peace – give peace
Pray for love – give love
Pray for Divine Light – give Divine Light

The alchemy of purification

The idea of purity might seem old fashioned in today's world. In yoga is it bound up with knowledge of our original goodness – That which is eternally pure in all.

At first we might experience parts of ourselves in conflict with finer qualities within us. But yoga does not advocate becoming guilty about the less refined parts of our nature, but to find ways in which we can harmonise the whole of ourselves and ground ourselves in the knowledge of the One Life that embraces all:

I purify myself and discover the Oneness that is every thing!

For me, the above affirmation sums up the essence of yoga – the discovery of our relationship with all that is; the knowing that God is in all life and all things, and all things – including ourselves – are united in God.

Jesus also reminds us of the importance of purity when he said, "Blessed are the pure in heart for they shall see God". Throughout the *Upanishads* the realisation of Brahman and its Oneness is expounded – the realisation of the individual self (*jivatman*) within the greater universal and Supreme Self (para-Brahman).

The eightfold yoga, as laid-out in Patanjali's *Sutra*, shows a way that can be used to experience this realisation. The initial stage is about purification through practising the daily life obligations of the *yamas* and *niyamas*, which help to purify and refine the mind (one of five sheaths/*koshas*) that envelopes the individual *atman*.

Let us then look at the five *koshas* as outlined in the *Taittiriya Upanishad*, and tie them in further with five of the eight-limbs of Patanjali's *Yoga Sutra* (practices that work with different facets of our being that can lead to a transcendence and a true embodiment of our finest qualities):

Five Koshas	Explanation	Yoga Sutra
Annamaya-kosha	Material or food sheath	*Asana*
Pranamaya-kosha	Subtle life force sheath	*Pranayama*
Manoma-kosha	Mind/sensory impressions sheath	*Concentration*
Vijnanamaya-kosha	Intellect: discerning and will sheath	*Meditation*
Anandamaya-kosha	Bliss sheath (closest to the *atman*)	*Samadhi*

It is seen that by working on all these levels, we understand the connectedness between our material and spiritual selves. But although transcendence is part of the path, it does not stop there, as physical life is included and seen as an important facet of spirituality in the majority of yogic paths.

The application of yogic practices is, therefore, seen as a way of purification, an integration of all parts of our being and a way to Self-realisation. The five sheaths Swami Adiswarananda reminds us, "may be compared to five different lamp-shades that obscure the effulgent Self within". By including and working on these different facets of ourselves we allow the light of our true Self to shine more brightly.

Study and meditate upon this ancient wisdom, but remember to apply and act upon the teachings in your life in order to live the *dharma* in all areas of existence. Use the whole of your life as a form of meditation and reflection for learning more about growth and awakening to the Divine, and make all your actions a method of dedication for unfolding your true spiritual nature. All this will lead you to knowledge of the Supreme Self that permeates all, and to an openness and freedom in everyday life. You have everything to gain and nothing to lose by becoming One with the All of eternal existence:

> *To allow sattva (purity) to grow in oneself*
> *one should nurture those things within you*
> *that are sattvic in nature.*
> *Only then will dharma become fixed within you.*
> *From that proceed to Self-realisation*
> *in which you once again know*
> *your own eternal and infinite nature.*
> Uddhava Gita

6

Where Everything Interconnects

SANTOSHAN

When the soul has lost her nature in the Oneness,
we can no longer speak of a 'soul', but of immeasurable Being.
MEISTER ECKHART

The essential abilities of mindfulness, insight and intuitive awareness function in ordinary everyday levels of consciousness, as well as in deeper and more profound states of knowing and awareness. In spiritual teachings, intuition and insight are associated more with the higher mind and supreme realisations of our true nature. But it is worth considering other ways they function. For example, intuition can be seen working at a physical, mental or emotional level. We might experience a physical pulling in the stomach area, a gut-feeling about something being right or wrong, or intuitively *know* or *feel* that something will happen.

We all experience insights into our life and work at some point or another, even if we are not following spiritual paths or practising meditative or contemplative disciplines. Artists and mediums both appear to have heightened intuitive awareness and are gifted with being able to tap into psychic and creative levels relatively easily. They may achieve this partly through heightened physical and feeling/emotional parts of themselves. Although knowledge gained purely through the physical senses is separate from intuitive knowledge, there are links where one springboards into the other. The word 'sensitive' used to describe mediums can also be seen to suggest this, as well as the practice of psychometry, which uses physical objects to psychically feel/tune into in order to gain intuitive information.

Ken Wilber implies that the psychic level is awakened to after intellectual maturity. However, not all seers, mediums or shamans who have access to the psychic realm are necessarily intellectuals. Though it can be argued that just as transcending the body does not imply becoming an Olympian athlete beforehand, so transcending the mind will equally not suggest developing it to the level of Plato or Einstein.

Nonetheless, the path is invariably not a linear one that moves systematically from the physical to the emotional, to the mental, to the psychic, to the Spirit or Supreme Self. We may move more predominantly from the body or feeling parts of ourselves and cultivate psychic awareness, then develop our intellectual powers at a later stage. The ride might be bumpier for doing so, but everyone's path will be different in some respect.

The word 'mindfulness' was chosen for *figure 3* in the *Love is Only Part of it* chapter, because of it being more commonly understood and used than the psychology term 'the observer'. Interestingly the Hindu yoga equivalent *sakshin* literally means 'observer', although it is usually translated as the 'witness consciousness'.

Levels of witness consciousness

The term witness consciousness can have wide connotations in yogic literature. From one perspective it links with the practice of mindfulness advocated by the Buddha, which has since become an indispensable part of the Buddhist tradition. It is a state of pure presence or bare awareness. Here it can be seen as a non-attached impersonal observer consciousness that is separate from the thinking mind; an inherent ability that we all possess, even though it may take time for us to properly become aware of it.

Witness consciousness focuses the mind, nourishes understanding, and allows us to stand-back and examine, in a non-attached and objective way, our actions, and inner and outer perceptions and to awaken to deeper levels of being. From its highest viewpoint, witness consciousness can refer to an essence of our Divine nature and Spirit, which transcends seer and seen reality: witnesser and witnessed (though sometimes associated with *purusha* when viewed from this perspective).

The two perspectives are generally not seen as separate from one another, but as One Reality functioning in different ways. Christian and Sufi mystics perform important practices, such as attentiveness, contemplative prayer and remembrance of God that tie in with ideas associated with the witness consciousness; for ultimately this is about awakening to the Divine's presence.

But it should be mentioned that mindfulness, awareness or the witness consciousness (whatever term you prefer) is not something we develop; it is the ability of noticing if we are aware of this facet of ourselves or not that is cultivated – what can paradoxically be called 'the practice of being aware of awareness', or 'aware of the mindful/ observer/witness consciousness'. In the supreme sense it is about pure Divine Consciousness and awareness.

At the level of everyday mindfulness, we become aware that our thoughts, feelings and physical experiences are constantly changing and ultimately transient. From this point we start the important process of owning, while also disidentifying from, impermanent parts of ourselves. We begin to notice and acknowledge how we work psychologically and how the entanglements of life cause us to lose sight of our spiritual nature. This leads us to cultivating wisdom and insight into ways that we can grow, accept day to day problems of life and reflect our authentic higher Self more purely.

It is an important stage, as development does not lie in solving all the hassles that life presents to us, but in acceptance, transcendence and in an integration of the whole of ourselves, which means doing something positive, such as surrendering to the greater perspective that the witness consciousness brings – a supporting peace, clarity and expansiveness – instead of fighting against or avoiding situations we find difficult to face.

When we are aware of this level of consciousness, we will notice that it remains unblemished by the events of life. Generally, we become caught up in the web of everyday existence and lose sight of this essential facet of ourselves that has the ability to silently stand-back and see the play of life with equanimous poise, and to live more freely, naturally and spontaneously in the present.

The realm of creative and psychic activity

This realm ties in with Carl Jung's concept of the collective unconscious, with the Cambridge biologist Rupert Sheldrake's morphogenic fields and resonance theories, with the domain of nature mysticism and with spiritual wisdom about Gaia and Mother Earth.

Additionally it links with our bodies, feelings and mind through the unconscious; although once this is realised it is obviously no longer an unconscious phenomenon. For we have to remember that development requires making aspects of the unconscious conscious, even though it is only our surface awareness that is in fact unconscious of other realms. Our true nature is not asleep and does not need waking-up. It is our surface consciousness that is in fact not fully awake or aware.

We can talk of various subtle grades of energy connected with this sphere, which link with different parts of ourselves, such as the higher mind and Spirit. Here we are moving away from ordinary stages of development and entering the field of transpersonal growth, which is beyond the individual/personal level of awareness.

There is plenty of food for thought regarding this. It is not only the territory of the medium, sharman, mystic, inspired artist, ancient or New Age Pagan, as the psychic part of us all connects us with this realm. Any form of visualisation or use of the imagination and intuition will imply tapping into creative and psychic forces. Just as the intellectual, emotional and physical parts of us function in various ways, there are numerous states and stages of development that apply to this area.

At a preliminary stage, the mind and emotions will more noticeably influence and colour experiences that are encountered here. One may not fully experience and become grounded in more abstract and higher states of pure bliss, pure peace or oneness, for example. The dualistic distinction between seer and seen reality will by no means be fully overcome. Bede Griffiths made the following observation about this:

> *As long as we are in the psychic world it is a world of multiplicity. There are many gods, many angels, many spirits, many powers of various sorts and this is why the psychic world is always somewhat ambiguous.*

None of this rules out the possibility that those embarking on a spiritual path will not touch higher states. The point is that they only *begin* here, and that they may not be fully and healthily integrated into the seeker's overall growth and become a firm stage of development. As Ken Wilber says, "States are free, but stages are earned". If there is a lack of individual work done, experience of psychic and creative energies *can* even lead to an unwholesome inflated ego personality.

Terms differ from teacher to teacher and many of them have their own interpretations. Because of its cosmic implications, the universal and omnipresent nature of the Divine can be seen to have strong associations with this realm of existence, and be perceived as a manifestation of the Divine standing in-between individualised being and the transcendent Absolute. But it will require superconscious awareness to have personal experience of this profound truth.

The Divine Mother Energy

From the Tantric yoga perspective, this level belongs to the world of Shakti: the creative Goddess/Mother energy that acts in and permeates all life in the cosmos, which is viewed as functioning in all physical and mental activity and as a source of infinite potential. It is to her that students of Tantra yoga seek to surrender, as well as to activate her power within themselves.

Modern science confirms that the universe is a sea of energy, and Christian mystics, such as Hildegard of Bingen, hold similar ideas to the yogic perspective:

> *The Earth is at the same time Mother,*
> *She is Mother of all that is natural,*
> *Mother of all that is human.*
> *She is Mother of all,*
> *For contained in her are the seeds of all.*

This ties in with Creation Spirituality. In some yoga teachings, everything, including the creative sound of *Om*, is seen to emerge from a cosmic form of *bindu* – a source point and centre of energy (comparable perhaps with the Big Bang theory) which also manifests individually within us – which structures itself into mathematical physical form. From *bindu* all the chakras emerge with their own energy centres and associated elements, forming and culminating in the creation of individualised existence and making our psychic being a microcosm of creative forces in the universe.

This realm was initially termed as *avyakta* (the matrix of nature), then *prakrti* (primordial nature), which in its lowest aspect is seen as the basic substance of material life and responsible for the appearance of many separate selves, causing misperceptions and blindness of our true interconnected nature. It was later expanded upon, probably because of the experiences of various yogis, by the introduction of Shakti.

Each progressive stage of development can be viewed as a diminishing degree of *prakrti's* baser influences and as an increase in awakening to our true spiritual Self. It is not so much a breaking in to a new awareness, but more of a developmental thinning out of what keeps us from realising and manifesting it.

Because Shakti connects with all parts of our being and is in constant interaction with the ultimate transcendent Divine Reality, it plays an important role in development. Through devotion or the path of spiritual knowledge, our feelings and thoughts can be lifted to higher states with the help of this energy. Through breathing exercises we become aware of the '*pranic* life force', which in Tantric teachings is viewed as a lower manifestation or instrument of Shakti, beneath the realm of consciousness.

Yoga teaches about the experience of *pranic* energy when our physical and mental energies are merged together, which can be seen to happen when we focus our attention on a particular part of the body. The fusion of mental and physical energy is also said to create the *pranic* sheath or energy body (discussed by Swamiji in chapters five and fifteen). *Prana* connects with, and is active in, libidinal-type drives and all activities of everyday life, including the personal will, moments of anger, altruistic actions, thoughts and desires and so on.

Through awareness of the flow of *pranic* energy and skilful mastery over ourselves, we can transform ways in which it interacts with our lives and become more gifted forces for good. The practice of '*prana* awareness' in this sense, though traditionally associated more with breath work, can be expanded to include mental and emotional development and therapeutic work. An essential in yoga, is to work towards purifying the mind and heart and the creative *pranic* life-force when it is functioning on a lower level.

But creative energy can be unpredictable and aspects of the unconscious need to be approached with care. That is why guidance is often needed to help us through various stages of unfoldment and is where the guru-student tradition of yoga plays an important role.

Likewise, it is also important to have a good supportive network of friends and helpers and a healthy environment for all areas of development and times of difficulty; for spirituality is multifaceted and needs to include individual and social growth, as well as cosmic levels of relating to the Divine. For those who have not read the rightly called classic of personal development, *The Stormy Search for the Self* by Christina and Stanislav Grof, cannot be recommended enough.

The process of spiritualising the whole of ourselves is done through the help of this energy emanating from the Divine Shakti. However, in Hindu wisdom, the Divine Mother can be associated both with gentle and nurturing qualities or with destructive aspects of her nature, although the latter is usually looked upon as symbolically helpful. For example, the Divine Mother in the form of Kali is believed to help devotees progress by severing their heads of ego. The Mother also has some associations with the word *maya*, which is often translated as illusion (in early teachings it only referred to creative power) and refers to the whole world being an illusion. But it can also be interpreted as delusion or misperceptions, i.e. as not seeing things as they really are, as a non-separate, interrelated Whole.

I think we have to be careful in the use of the word illusion, as it can imply and justify a lack of concern for life and others, whereas a true realisation of oneness and non-separateness leads to realising our interrelationship with all and our responsibilities for the Earth and its inhabitants.

Superconsciousness

For many writers on development, superconsciousness can refer to all kinds of higher and expanded states. In Yogananda's writings on the *Bhagavad Gita* he mentions various stages of superconsciousness, including hearing astral sounds, seeing visions, experiencing *pranic* and cosmic energy, which lead to the realisation of God's omnipresence and beyond. The founder of Psychosynthesis psychology, Roberto Assagioli, also placed a wide range of abilities and qualities under its heading, including acts of heroism.

As a help to identify some higher and lower states and stages of awakening they could be listed under the following two headings:

1. TRANSPERSONAL CONSCIOUSNESS (BEYOND INDIVIDUAL AWARENESS) OR LOWER SUPERCONSCIOUSNESS (CREATIVE AND PSYCHIC ACTIVITY)

Lower and higher levels of intuitive insight and psychic and spiritual awareness that connect with moments of inspiration, creativity and lower influences of Shakti, as well as with *prana* and an element of the omnipresent universal Divine Consciousness (cosmic consciousness/higher Shakti) – an evolving transcendence and opening to states and stages beyond the thinking mind and ordinary sensory awareness.

2. HIGHER SUPERCONSCIOUSNESS

Higher levels of spiritual consciousness and intuitive insight that lead to a purer awakening to the omnipresent universal Divine, and to glimpses and knowledge of the Supreme Self as the Ultimate Transcendent Absolute – realisations of pure bliss, pure being and pure consciousness.

Superconsciousness can be seen as acting as an intermediate level between higher and lower levels, and as a facet of witness consciousness, expanding beyond ordinary awareness of the mind and senses. Through it we are drawn to and attain ultimate knowledge of ourselves, our relationship with everything and everyone, the connectednesss of all life, and discover the transcendent Reality beyond all manifest forms and relative experience.

It is a level of awareness that opens the way to wisdom, compassion, peace, unity and supreme insight into our nature. At its greatest, it is a pure state and includes realms of unfoldment that lead to the Divine in Its immanent, omnipresent and highest aspects.

Whereas the psychic and creative level can be unpredictable, higher superconsciousness leads to the discovery of our finest attributes (*sattvic* qualities). When actualised, it can help us to bring about stability, clarity and equanimity, and a transformation and harmonisation of any conflicting parts into a balanced and sacred whole.

In the higher superconscious, qualities that emanate from the Supreme Self and reflect the true nature of our being are found in abundance. Such teachings are found not only in yoga and Vedanta philosophy, where the Divine with attributes (Saguna Brahman) is recognised – although different terms for superconscious might be used – but also in contemporary spiritual psychologies, such as Psychosynthesis.

In comparison, Christian theology and mysticism sees God as the Eternal Good. Holiness, which is a comparable word to wholeness, is achieved by opening to the presence of the Divine at the centre of our being, and allowing Its mystery to heal and lead us to completeness.

What is unique in Sri Aurobindo's writings, is his idea about the 'supermind' (a supreme superconscious phenomenon and projection of the Divine); though he believed it was mentioned in the *Rig Veda* and the *Upanishads* as *'vijnana'* (liberating knowledge and consciousness). For him, the supermind stands above all other states of knowing and evolvement, uninhibited by *prakrti* and restrictive levels of consciousness. Because of its status, he calls it the 'truth Consciousness', which leads to a transcendent gnosis through which higher knowledge is revealed.

A crucial point he makes is that in the final stages of development we do not realise the Divine from a state of distorted partial knowledge, but from a level of unafflicted consciousness. We start from truth and light and continue in truth and light. We move from clear perceptions to deeper perceptions; from a growing expansiveness to awakening to the Divine in Its purest form – which is without form.

Sri Aurobindo saw the supermind as an extension of the Ultimate, eternally acting in and supporting the universe and leading humankind to its evolutionary spiritual fulfilment. The 'Omega point' of the French priest, mystic and paleontologist Teilhard de Chardin corresponds almost identically with Sri Aurobindo's teachings about the supermind. Both taught about the Divine Consciousness penetrating Creation and integrating all in a final stage of transcendence. They both pointed out how at every stage a lower level of consciousness is transcended, it is also integrated into a higher one.

But as well as transcendence and integration, Sri Aurobindo's yoga is about an embodiment of higher levels. His writings show that a complete change cannot be brought about unless the higher planes of existence are allowed to descend and transform our individual nature.

This point is also made by the contemporary American psychologist John Welwood, who mentions that along with transcendent realisations, we also need to embody our experiences and integrate them into our everyday lives, and so reflect and manifest the Highest within us.

The interconnected Self and unitive states of consciousness

All previous stages can, to a certain degree, be easily talked about. But under this heading, things become more difficult, as it is about an awakening to existence that cannot really be expressed by language or grasped by conceptual thought, because to conceptualise or express it is to limit it.

Probably in an attempt to avoid conceptualisation and the limitations of language, the Buddha promoted the idea of awakening to neither self nor no-self (to self-less-ness). To an extent his approach is shared by others, that in the deepest realms of being there is no distinction between the 'I' and the 'not I'.

It is the non-dual Reality that mystics of various traditions remind us of, where the traces of our separate selves are overcome. In Christian mysticism it is the Unitive Consciousness where the ultimate mystery is realised and the seeker recognises his or her co-relationship with the Creator:

> ... it is the intimate union in the depths of your own heart, of God's spirit and your own secret inmost self, so that you and He are in all truth One Spirit.
> THOMAS MERTON

Although the Buddha observed a noble silence about Absolute realms

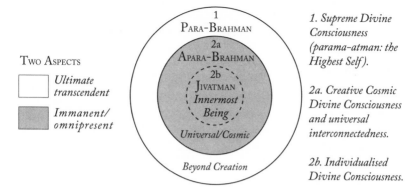

FIGURE 4: *Interconnected Gradations of the Divine.*

of awakening, the realisation of non-separateness and peacefulness are essential facets of his teachings on enlightenment. For Mahayana Buddhists, exterior and interior existence is One Taste and Reality that is always present. Our eternal Buddha nature, which is twofold – developable and naturally abiding within us – transcends thought, is thoroughly pure, undefiled, empty of all dualities and experienced as a joyous expansiveness with infinite positive potential.

The Spirit, the true Self or *atman* in non-dual Hindu yoga is seen to have no distinction from the Divine (Brahman) and is connected with two aspects of It: passive and active – one which, the *Upanishads* tell us, stands outside time, Creation and causality and supports the whole cosmos (an ultimate transcendent aspect); and a second, which refers to the true and same Being in all (a universal and individualised aspect).

In Hindu philosophy the terms *para* and *apara* are used to describe these different perspective (see *figure 4*). They are also used to describe higher and lower aspects of Shakti and *prakrti*. Our innermost Divine essence has associations with the *jivatman*, which is sometimes seen as 'the soul' (a sticky term at the best of times as everyone appears to have a different interpretation of it). These are all different vantage points of One Reality acting in and transcending the universe. The analogy of a hologram is sometimes used to demonstrate this One in all and all in One. If a hologram is broken into pieces, each fragment will still hold the original image.

Ultimately, as in Buddhism, there is no interior or exterior. By recognising the Divine within, we come to recognise the Divine which is in everything and how everything is ultimately in the Divine. In a passage from the *Crest-Jewel of Wisdom* attributed to Shankara, a student gives a moving account of awakening to the Brahman-*atman* relationship:

> *My mind fell like a hailstone into that vast expanse of Brahman's ocean. Touching one drop of it, I melted away and became one with Brahman. And now, though I return to human consciousness, I abide in the joy of the Atman....*
>
> *Here is the ocean of Brahman, full of endless joy. How can I accept or reject anything? Is there anything apart or distinct from Brahman?*
>
> *Now, finally and clearly, I know that I am the Atman, whose nature is eternal joy. I see nothing, I hear nothing, I know nothing that is separate from me.*

This passage confirms the findings of the early *Upanishads*, which are about realising an Ultimate Oneness and discovering that those who know the *atman* also know Brahman, the Supreme Ground of all. Similarly the New Testament reminds us, "In this One we live and move and have our being". But we need to remember that Brahman is not a part of us – we are a part of Brahman. Everything has its origins in this Reality. It is the Source of all knowledge and wisdom – revealed by identity – and Power behind all activity. It is described as *sat-chit-ananda* (pure Being, pure Consciousness and pure Bliss) and as immanent and transcendent by various yogis and mystics.

Although the *Upanishads*, like all mystical traditions, display pantheistic leanings about the omnipresence of Divinity, sections show they also point to panentheism – a Divinity that is both in and beyond the created universe. Similarly, Christian mystics, such as St. Symeon, remind us that, "For those who look with their physical eyes, God is nowhere to be seen. For those who contemplate Him in spirit, He is everywhere. He is in all, yet beyond all".

For Sri Aurobindo, active Divine Will and Intelligence are forces of pure Consciousness (*chit*) and Divine Love is seen as another aspect of pure Bliss (*ananda*). Technically we cannot talk about qualities that the Absolute/highest aspect of the Divine possesses, or of It being a state or stage of development – just as the highest aspect of ourselves cannot be reduced to these terms. Perhaps the closest description that anyone has given is to say that the Divine simply *is*.

Three levels of reality

There are three basic levels of awareness shown below that fit with various beliefs and models and link with *figures 3* and *4*. For a developmental model that starts from early childhood we can add the 'pre-personal' stage that Ken Wilber mentions. The body, feelings and mind, though intrinsically bound-up with spiritual and transpersonal unfoldment, are chiefly the territory of individual development, which then moves into transpersonal growth (a realm housing states of awareness beyond the restrictions of personal identity) and the realisation of the Supreme Self. A complete transformation will obviously not come about unless all levels are in tune and harmonised with one another.

DEVELOPMENTAL MODEL
1a. Pre-personal
1b. Personal
2. Transpersonal
3. Supreme Self
   (authentic nature)

MYSTICAL MODEL
1. Individual
2. Universal (creative)
3. Transcendent Absolute (pure)

THREEFOLD YOGIC MODEL
1. Finite/gross body
2. Subtle/psychic body
3. Causal body

PART TWO
Exercises

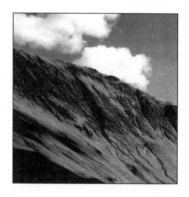

May we all continue to evolve into the Divine Light.
SWAMI DHARMANANDA

*There is no stage where the spiritual journey comes to its end,
as the path is an ever-expanding spiral in which
there are many awakenings along the way.*
SANTOSHAN

O you, in quest of God, you seek Him everywhere,
You verily are the God, not apart from Him!
Already in the midst of the boundless ocean,
Your quest resembles the search of a drop for the ocean!
DARA SHIKOH

… meditation is to allow God's mysterious and silent presence within us
to become more and more the reality of our lives.
JOHN MAIN

We don't use concentration to run away from our suffering.
We concentrate to make ourselves deeply present.
When we walk, stand, or sit in concentration,
people can see our stability and stillness.
Living each moment deeply, sustained concentration comes naturally,
and that, in turn, gives rise to insight.
Right concentration leads to happiness, and it also leads to right action.
The higher our degree of concentration, the greater the quality of our life.
THICH NHAT HANH

Let your mind be quiet,
realising the beauty of the world,
and the immense boundless treasures that it holds in store.
EDWARD CARPENTER

Just as rivers flow from east and west to merge with the one sea,
forgetting that they were ever separate rivers,
so all beings lose their separateness when they eventually merge into pure being.
CHANDOGYA UPANISHAD

7

Practices on the Breath

SWAMI DHARMANANDA

Homage to the Breath of Life, for this whole universe obeys it …
… O Breath of Life, turn not thy back on me;
None other than I shalt thou be.
As an embryo in the waters, so I within myself
Bind thee, that I may live!

ATHARVA VEDA

The exercises in this chapter, and in chapter 15, should be undertaken with an awareness of one's own physical capabilities – working with breath awareness and, as far as this chapter is concerned, coordination of the breath with movement. Take care not to over-extend in either the stretching or the breathing.

Although these exercises can help people with heart disease, high blood pressure, arthritis or suffering from symptoms of stress, work with care, and take note of the general precautions below before trying any of the exercises in this book.

General Precautions

All the practices mentioned in this book are suitable for most people of all age groups. However, if unsure about the suitability of any exercise, seek professional advice, such as a person who is expertly trained in these practices or a knowledgeable doctor. There should be no strain, either physically or mentally. Care should be taken not to hyperventilate. No retention, especially of the in-breath with high blood pressure or heart problems. No retention of the out-breath with low blood pressure. Care must be taken not to over-extend the breath with a hiatus hernia.

81

HARMONISING BREATH

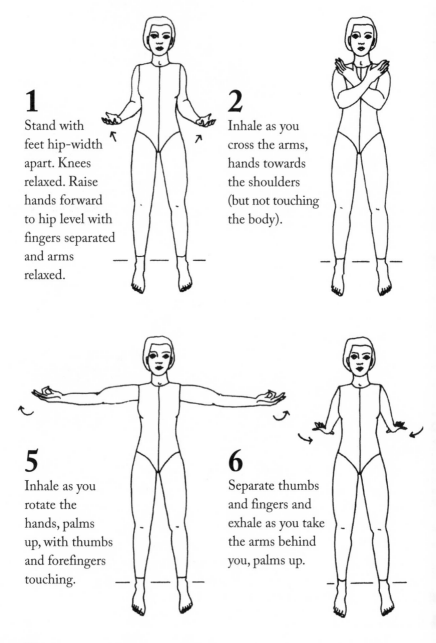

1
Stand with feet hip-width apart. Knees relaxed. Raise hands forward to hip level with fingers separated and arms relaxed.

2
Inhale as you cross the arms, hands towards the shoulders (but not touching the body).

5
Inhale as you rotate the hands, palms up, with thumbs and forefingers touching.

6
Separate thumbs and fingers and exhale as you take the arms behind you, palms up.

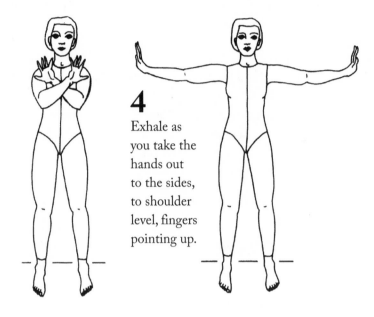

3

Turn the
palms
forward.

4

Exhale as
you take the
hands out
to the sides,
to shoulder
level, fingers
pointing up.

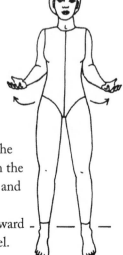

7

Inhale as
you turn the
arms from the
shoulders and
scoop the
hands forward
to hip level.

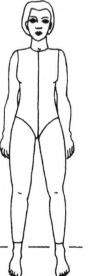

8

Exhale as you
relax the arms
to the sides.
*Practise 3-5
times before any
meditation
practices.*

MEDITATIVE BREATH

Sit quietly in a comfortable posture – an easy crossed leg posture or in a chair. To assist a stable, relaxed, well-balanced posture, and to avoid strain on the lower back and knees, it is suggested that you sit on a *firm* cushion or on a telephone directory, but sit towards the edge of these – not too far back. Take time to make sure that you are comfortably seated and become aware of the steadiness of your posture.

1. Become aware of the breath, and the temperature of the breath, cool breath on the inhalation, slightly warmer on the exhalation. Continue with this observation for a few moments.

2. Become aware of the depth and the rhythm of the breath.

3. After a few moments, become aware of the breath flowing in and the breath flowing out.

4. Take 10 breaths in this way, mentally repeating, 'The breath is flowing in, the breath is flowing out'.

5. Now become aware of the in-breath only – your awareness should be focused on the in-breath, just allowing the out-breath to happen (10 breaths).

6. Then change and focus your awareness on the out-breath only, allowing the in-breath to take care of itself (10 breaths).

7. Then become aware once more of the natural flow of the in-and out-breath for 5 – 10 minutes.

8. Gently stretch, bringing your awareness back to the outside world.

8

Affirming our True Nature

SANTOSHAN

The following relaxation exercise will help relax and heal the mind, body, feelings and emotions and place you in a responsive state for meditation practice.

1. Sit in a quiet place, where you will not be disturbed. Sit with your eyes closed in your preferred meditation position, keeping the spine erect.

2. Mentally check for any tension in the body, starting with the feet and slowly work your way up to the top of the head. Be aware of any tension being held in any part of the body, paying particular attention to the neck, shoulder and facial areas. Smile then relax the smile. As you go from one area to another, mentally say to yourself, 'I liberate my . . . (name the part) from any tension', with the out-breath, and be calmly aware of all tension leaving the body as you do this.

This whole exercise should take approximately 5 to 10 minutes. Once you have completed this exercise, mentally or vocally say to yourself, 'My whole body is liberated and free and totally relaxed'.

When you have finished the exercise, be quiet for a moment then repeat the following affirmation:

> *I am aware of the Divine as the one creative and loving force that permeates all. I acknowledge Its creativity and compassion as the ultimate ground of my being. I know of no limitation in my life and awaken to a world of infinite co-creative possibilities with the Divine. I am an open and a receptive channel for truth, love, harmony, goodness and wisdom and manifest these in me now.*

As the eternal Spirit has no boundaries, there is nothing I cannot achieve, accept or overcome. All is in tune with my life. I am at peace with all that surrounds me. I see through all existence and am continuously aware of the Divine's presence in every moment and every action.

The humming breath

Sit in your chosen meditation position with the spine erect. Close your eyes and gently inhale a deep breath. Now gently close your ears with your index fingers without applying too much pressure and make a smooth and continuous 'm' sound as you slowly exhale. Do not over extend the out-breath any more than it feels comfortable.

Repeat this exercise 3 to 5 times. As you breathe out, gently make an 'm' sound. Be aware of its sound vibrating within your body and the space around you. This exercise helps to relax and to focus the mind and to revitalise the body in a soothing way. Yogis say that if you practise this exercise regularly your voice will become sweet and beautiful to listen to.

When you have finished the exercise, be quiet for a moment then repeat the following affirmation:

I am at one with the infinite, wise and compassionate Self. I release all discord and inhibiting patterns from my life. I am a pure representative of eternal good, and practise harmlessness in all thoughts, words and deeds. I respect the equality of life and take pleasure in its abundant and creative diversity. I am open and true to myself and others – selfless and skilful in all activities – and immerse the whole of my being into virtuous living, making all actions for the emergence of spiritual awareness and the realisation of the interconnected universal Self.

Meditation on the interrelatedness of life

The following meditation incorporates the creative use of the imagination and can help to bring the whole of you into balance – body, mind, emotions and Spirit. It takes approximately 25 minutes to practise.

Because the practice is fairly long and detailed, you may like to ask a friend to lead you through it or record yourself reading it and meditate to your recording. Be sure to leave an appropriate length of space between each part if you do this. Step 1 is a preliminary settling down stage, which briefly focuses on some things that are incorporated as specific stages in the exercise.

1. Relax and breathe normally, slowly and rhythmically, keeping the spine erect. Close your eyes. Become aware of the body. Feel its weight on the chair or cushion you are sitting on. Think about the body and its relation to the Earth and the universe, and how it is made of atoms that are the building blocks of all physical life that once made stars, plants and other life in the universe.

Become aware of the breath as it enters in and out of the body. Realise that every breath you take feeds the plants and in return their oxygen feeds you. Reflect upon your interconnectedness with all life and nature. Notice if the sun passes behind clouds and makes a difference to the brightness of the place you are sitting in.

Listen to any sounds of nature that can be heard around you – the rustling of leaves in the wind, the singing of birds, the humming or buzzing of insects, the pattering of rain or the trickling of a running stream. Feel the natural vibration of nature, and feel yourself at one and in harmony with it. Stay with your feelings, thoughts and observations for a while.

2. As you breathe in, mentally say to yourself, 'I breathe in the stabilising earth element'. As you breathe out, mentally repeat, 'I breathe out the stabilising earth element'. Repeat this five times.

As you repeat the words, feel the earth's strength entering and connecting with your body – balancing and harmonising all of your body's organs, and making every part of you function optimally, as well as rhythmically with itself and other facets of your being. Feel it healing and grounding the whole of your physical self, bringing strength and vitality. Stay with this element for a while.

3. Become aware of the breath and as you breathe in mentally say to yourself, 'I breathe in the soothing water element'. As you breathe out mentally repeat, 'I breathe out the soothing water element'. Repeat this five times.

As you repeat the words, remember that water is the elixir of all physical life. Feel the soothing effect of the water element gently replenishing you and feel its calming influence. Know that it has the power to restore and refresh your whole being and balance all parts. Stay with this element for a while.

4. Become aware of the breath and as you breathe in, mentally say to yourself, 'I breathe in the rejuvenating sun element'. As you breathe out, mentally repeat, 'I breathe out the rejuvenating sun element'. Repeat this five times.

As you repeat the words, feel the purifying and comforting effects of the sun element transforming you and refining all inhibiting emotions, feelings and thoughts. Realise that all human life requires warmth to be truly alive and how this warmth and energy comes ultimately from the sun, which gives life to plants which feed you and other life on Earth. Realise it is helping you to let go of all concerns and be more peacefully present in the eternal now of existence and the radiance of eternal goodness. Stay with this element for a while.

5. Become aware of the breath and as you breathe in, mentally say to yourself, 'I breathe in the cleansing air element'. As you breathe out mentally say, 'I breathe out the cleansing air element'. Do this five times.

As you repeat the words, feel the cleansing and inspiring effect of the air element. Feel a clearness of the mind and a relaxing of the body and the emotions. Know that this element is restoring your mind, body, feelings and emotions to health and perfect balance with all existence. Stay with this element for a while.

6. Become aware of the breath and as you breathe in, mentally say to yourself, 'I breathe in the expansive space element' (often termed 'ether' in spiritual literature). As you breathe out, mentally say, 'I breathe out the expansive space element'. Do this five times.

As you repeat the words, feel your mind, consciousness and whole being expanding. Feel this element awakening you to the authentic Self and harmonising all parts. Feel it embracing and enveloping you and lifting your consciousness to a higher level of existence.

Feel this element permeating everything within you and around you. Know that within this element you may find time to rest, restore and replenish your whole being – your body, mind and emotions. Stay with this element for a while.

7. Become aware of the breath and as you breathe in, mentally say to yourself, 'I breathe in the loving-presence of the infinite Self'. As you breathe out, mentally say, 'I breathe out the loving-presence of the infinite Self'. Do this five times. Feel all that is pure and good in life. Feel peace, love, joy, light, beauty and harmony. Know that you are a pure manifestation of the Divine Spirit. Awaken to and manifest this Divinity within you now, and let it shine through and permeate your whole being. Stay with this experience for a while and strengthen your awareness of it.

8. Slowly become aware of your surroundings and collect your thoughts and then repeat the follow affirmation:

> *I awaken to the compassionate Spirit in all. I am aware of the Divine's sacred power working in me, through me and around me. I acknowledge the Divine's omnipresent goodness, and allow it to transform and radiate through my whole being – bringing all areas of my life into harmony and loving unity with others.*

PART THREE
The Great Paths of Yoga

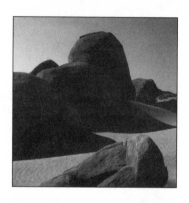

*May the rays of the Divine Spirit shine upon you
and may you grow in beauty and love.*
SWAMI DHARMANANDA

*Spiritual growth is the emergence of a pure mind and heart
filled with wisdom and compassion.*
SANTOSHAN

Love is patient; love is kind; love is not envious or boastful or arrogant or rude.
It does not insist on its own way; it is not irritable or resentful;
it does not rejoice in wrongdoing, but rejoices in the truth.
CORINTHIANS

Blessed are the man and woman who have grown beyond their greed
and have put an end to their hatred and no longer nourish illusions.
PSALMS

Yoga allows you to achieve a sense of wholeness in your life, where you do not
feel like you are constantly trying to fit the broken pieces together.
B. K. S. IYENGAR

The gift of truth is more precious than all other gifts.
The taste of truth is sweeter than all other tastes.
The joy of truth surpasses all other joys.
The loss of desires conquers all suffering.
DHAMMAPADA

Joy Comes from God …
From joy all beings have come,
by joy they all live,
and unto joy they all return.
TAITTIRIYA UPANISHAD

To lead a life of truth, beauty, and virtue,
we must use our minds without discrimination or duality,
perceiving things as they are
and treating all sentient beings as inherently equal.
MASTER HSING YUN

9

Sanctity of Mantra

SWAMI DHARMANANDA

Mantra Yoga utilises the power of sound as a method of inducing introspection and subtle mental changes, and to invoke mental and psychic manifestations.
SWAMI SATYANANDA

If used correctly mantra is a sure way towards understanding and achieving knowledge of the spiritual Self. It is a tool that can focus our awareness with full protection and liberates us from chaotic thought-waves of the mind. Today many people in the West are more aware of mantra and its uses than ever before. The pioneering work of the English Benedictine monk John Main, who was introduced to Eastern meditation by Swami Sivananda, has led numerous Christians to use the ancient Aramaic prayer 'Maranatha' (Come Lord) as a form of mantra practice.

In the book *Christian Yogic Meditation* by Father Amaldas, he writes about using *Om Nama Christaya* (prostrations to the Lord Jesus Christ) as a mantra practice, and others that can be used, such as *Yeshu Yeshu Yeshuve* (Jesus, Jesus, Jesus) and *Yeshu Yeshu Jai Jai Abba* (Glory to Jesus, glory to the Father). The Eastern Christian practice of using the Jesus Prayer, where one verbally or mentally repeats 'Lord Jesus Christ have mercy upon me' with each breath, has also been adopted by Christian contemplatives in the West.

There are many types of mantras available on CD, and these are becoming popular for relaxation and stress release. In some cases this is leading to further enquiry about meditation practices and mantra for spiritual development. But perhaps a little more knowledge regarding mantra would not go amiss.

Mantra, kirtan and japa

Kirtan is the singing or chanting of the names of the Divine Lord – giving praise to God. This practice is usually performed at the end of other practices. It is said to release and liberate excess energy. Chanting in unison is slightly different and has a different effect and is usually practised in the morning or before meditation to focus the mind.

Japa is the repetition of a mantra. This can be a seed (*bija*) mantra, which I will describe later, or a deity mantra (a mantra chanted to a particular God, such as Shiva, Krishna or the Mother). *Japa* is considered to be one of the most direct ways to Self-realisation, as it is said to be able to remove the impurities that mask the spiritual light and truth within us.

Usually the mantra used would be a meditative mantra, which is often used to help dispel the darkness of ignorance. Swami Sivananda says in his book *The Practice of Yoga* that, "The efficiency of the Japa is accentuated according to the degree of concentration. The mind should be fixed on the source. Then only will you realise the maximum benefits of a Mantra".

For those who wish to practise *japa* and do not have a mantra, the use of *So-ham* is advised (mentally repeat *So* on the inhalation and *ham* on the exhalation). I know that I have previously referred to it in this book, but as this chapter is specifically about mantra it also needs to be mentioned here. This mantra, known as the breath mantra, is suitable for all students and means 'I am That', which can be interpreted as 'I am a spark of the Divine that is both within and beyond all existence'.

It is said that with every breath we take the *So-ham* mantra is manifest, so this is obviously a very practical mantra to use. If you are not already practising *japa*, this can be a good one to start with. If you are prepared to experiment, you will eventually find a form of mantra practice that will be suitable for you.

The role of mantra

Mantra is an important part of yoga. It plays a large part in the practice of bhakti yoga, the yoga of devotion. Chanting or singing hymns of devotion – no matter what religion – helps to bring about a deeper awareness of our relationship with the sacred and with the

Divine that permeates all.

In Patanjali's *Yoga Sutra*, mantra is part of his system for enlightenment. Sutra 17 of chapter 3 states, "By making *samyama* on the sound of the Word (*Om*), one's perception of its meaning, and one's reaction to it, one obtains understanding of all sounds uttered by beings". The word *samyama* refers to a combination of concentration (*dharana*), meditation (*dhyana*) and meditative absorption (*samadhi)*, through which one attains freedom from conditioned worldly existence (*samsara*).

Mantra is a creative instrument that can help us in our development. It is a force, as is all sound, which is a vibration and gives rise to definite forms. St. John's Gospel reminds us of this in the opening passage: "In the beginning was the Word ..."

As sound mantra can be constructive/creative or destructive. What caused the walls of Jericho to fall? Therefore, remember that mantra should be used with the right attitude of mind.

The effect of sound is such that certain mantras and devotional songs (*ragas*) are only performed at particular times of the day, as it is accepted that different times, such as sunrise and sunset, have different vibrations and energies. It is said that the Vedic teachings – which includes the *Upanishads* – have 'inner meaning' and should be verbally quoted. This indicates that the intonation and metre of certain words can be used as a method for discovering the inner wisdom of these teachings. This is something that is often overlooked, and reminds us that just silently reading the *Vedas* can neglect an important facet of their power.

Seed mantras

Bija mantras means 'seed mantras' in English. Swami Radha poetically wrote about them in the following passage:

> *Each Mantra has a bija or seed. This is the essence of the Mantra and it gives the Mantra its special power – its self-generating power. Just as within a seed is hidden a tree, so the energy in the Mantra is the seed from which all will grow a beautiful spiritual being.*

Not only do the chakras have associated seed mantras, but also each has a particular note/sound making a musical scale. The different pitch (*swara*) and form (*varma*) of each note will have different effects on the nervous system and consciousness. Some seed mantras have subtle meanings which are not conveyed openly. In connection with the chakras, we have the 'five great elements' (*mahabhutas*), of which each have their own seed mantra:

SEED MANTRA	DESCRIPTION
Lam	*Prithivi* (earth)
Vam	*Apa* (water)
Ram	*Agni* (fire)
Yam	*Vayu* (air)
Ham	*Akasha* (ether)

The great elements mantras are said to activate the various elements existing within man and woman, according to the method of repetition given by the guru.

The elements and every deity have their own seed letter (*bija-akshara*). Strictly speaking a seed mantra consists of a single letter. For example, the letter R (*ra* sound) in the yogic tradition represents one of

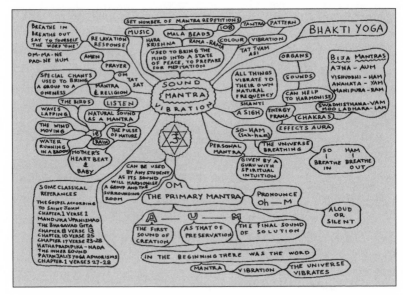

FIGURE 5: *Organic Note-taking.*

the five great elements, namely fire. But the seed mantra is pronounced as 'Ram', as a consonant cannot be pronounced without a vowel. Hence the 'ra' sound as mentioned above, but with an added 'm'.

The 'm' is known as the termination of the vowel. It is sounded with a particular form of nasal breathing done in yoga (termed *candra-bindu*), which has links with the Absolute manifestation of sound (*nada*) within us and the universe.

Practices of mantra

Mantra repetition can be performed in several ways, such as verbal repetition (*vaikhari japa*), whispered repetition (*upamshu japa*) or mental repetition (*manasika japa*).

Even writing with mental repetition (*likhita japa*) is a form of mantra practice, as the words are still being repeated in one's mind. Organic note-taking during a lecture or talk on mantra can also be viewed as a form of practice. Done with the right frame of mind it can prove to be just as effective as any other form of mantra practice. The illustration on the opposite page by one of my students is an example of what I mean by organic note-taking.

Swami Sivananda described mantra practice as, "A sacred word or syllable, or set of words, through the repetition and reflection of which one attains perfection or realisation of the Self". We can only know this through experience, so we can only know by practising some form of mantra.

The healing power of mantra

The therapeutic value of mantra is in bringing the four elements – earth, water, fire, air and ether – into equipoise. It is generally considered in Ayurvedic and Chinese medicine that when the four elements within us are working in harmony with one another, our health and body's energies will be synchronised and balanced.

The rhythmical vibrations of the mantra are seen to regulate unsteady vibrations of the various sheaths (*koshas*) connected to the individual. They also help to clear any blockages in our energy flow.

Although seed mantras have no literal meaning in themselves, they can have significant inner, subtle implications. When used, spiritual awareness can be heightened, which aids the holistic healing process of harmonising our bodies, minds, feelings and Spirit. If we consider the power of *Om* – the Word of Creation – then why should we doubt the power of sound and mantra to have healing properties? In Swami Sivananda's excellent *Science of Yoga* series he states:

> *Chronic disease can be cured by Mantra. Chanting of Mantras generates potent spiritual waves, or divine vibrations. Mantras remove the root cause of suffering. They fill the cells with pure Sattva, or divine energy. They destroy the microbes and vivify the cells and tissues.*

As mentioned, sounds are vibrations. Amazingly they also create different shapes. Scientific studies have shown how notes produced by the voice and certain instruments can be traced-out on a tray of sand and produce distinctive geometrical shapes, such as waves or circular patterns.

I have seen a similar experiment using equipment such as an oscilloscope. Various patterns were created by using varied notes and note combinations. The mantra *Om*, when chanted with the correct vibration, produced a perfect circle. Therefore, support can be given to the yogic belief that sounds create shapes. If sound can do this, then it would appear that sound may also have the power to change the shape of molecules and should, therefore, have the potential to bring about changes in health.

Further support for sound in healing is given by the use of ultrasonic and infrasonic treatment by medical practitioners in clinics and hospitals and by many physiotherapists treating sports injuries. Music is being used in many cases, including the treatment of cancer in order to bring about a state of relaxation that can aid the healing process.

Recent research into music therapy has dramatically helped some children with Asperger's syndrome (a mild autistic disorder that is more common in boys) to connect and relate more with and understand others, and express themselves and communicate in an increased natural way. The therapist plays a piano and sings in various ways that highlight – through changing keys, volume and rhythm – the child's moods, which helps him or her to get more in touch with and understand his or her emotions and how to interact with others. The results in some cases have been quite remarkable.

The chanting of certain mantras can be used to bring about a feeling of inner peace and well being. It can bring calmness to an over active or a troubled mind, or an unbalanced physical body. This in itself is an important element of healing.

There are some mantras, when repeated in certain ways, are credited with healing powers for specific diseases. Some of the vowels are said to stimulate areas of the body. The *Maha-mritunjaya* mantra (*Om trayambakam yajamahe sugandhim pushtivardhanam, urvarukamiva bandhanaan, mrityor muskshiya maamritaat*) is considered an extremely powerful healing and protective mantra and translates as the following:

> *We worships the three-eyed Lord (Shiva) of excellent fragrance, the increaser of welfare. Just as the cucumber from its binding/vine may be released from death, not from immortality.*

However, we must always remember that mantra needs to be used with care, or adverse conditions can be created, as it may awaken energies that we are not ready to handle. We are, after all, using a powerful tool that can bring about great changes in spiritual development. So we must proceed gently and wisely in mantra practice.

The sacred sound of *Om*

> *The subtle energies of the body spread like spokes from a hub,*
> *And where they meet, there is found the all-supporting Brahman.*
> *Realise the Self as Om. Thus may you safely cross the waters of*
> *darkness and reach the farther shore of light.*
> MUNDAKA UPANISHAD

The greatest of all seed mantras is the *Pranava*: the *Om* mantra. It is the most powerful of all mantras, the symbol – or sound – of Creation and Brahman, the Supreme Absolute/God. *Om* contains and is considered as the seed of all the other *bija* mantras. It is the sound from which all other sounds emanate. The *Mandukya Upanishad* reminds us that, "*Om* the imperishable Sound, is the Seed of all that exists".

According to the ancient teachings of the *Vedas* and the *Upanishads*, *Om* is the primordial sound from which the whole universe was created, is sustained by and into which it will eventually dissolve.

The sound of *Om* is seen as the basis of all sound, consisting of three components: *A*, *U* and *M*. Together these encompass all sound vibrations. Swami Vivekananda reminds about this:

> *The first letter A, is the root sound, the key, pronounced without touching any part of the tongue or palate; M represents the last sound in the series, being produced with closed lips, and the U rolls from the very root to the end of the sounding-board of the mouth. Thus, Om represents the whole phenomena of sound-producing.*

Significance of the three sounds of *Om*

The three sounds of *Om* represent different trinities. For example:

Three aspects of time – *past, present and future.*
Three aspects of existence – *birth, life and death.*
Three aspects of being – *body, mind and spirit.*
Three aspects of Divinity – *creation, preservation and destruction.*

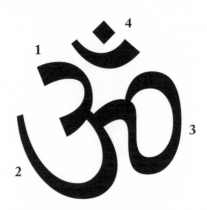

FIGURE 6: *Om.*

The three aspects of Divinity are sometimes assigned individually to Brahma the creator, Vishnu the preservation and Shiva the destroyer. Collectively termed the 'Trimurti'. However, Brahma, Vishnu and Shiva can individually be accredited with having all three aspects. The three sounds of *Om* also have associations with the three *gunas*: purity and light (*sattva guns*), action and energy (*ragas guna*) and inertia and darkness (*tamas guna*).

The actual symbolic representation of *Om* is seen to represent three ordinary states of consciousness: (1) dreamless sleep, (2) wakefulness and (3) dreaming. The crescent moon and dot (4) represents the Supreme Reality and liberation from conditioned worldly existence.

A symbol for the Ultimate

As stated, *Om* signifies God who/which transcends the limitations of time, existence, being, the three aspects of divinity, the *gunas* and three states of consciousness. It also represents a fourth state – pure consciousness – where individual, universal and transcendent levels of consciousness merge into One. It is a level of consciousness that leads to an awakening and a realisation of the Divine in Its omnipresent and absolute form.

The chanting of *Om* sets up powerful vibrations which can be felt throughout our entire being, which can affect our body, our mind and our psyche. Chanting *Om* calms and concentrates the mind and helps to make it one-pointed and focused. It is energising, stabilising, exhilarating, strengthening, inspiring and cheering – let us not forget that yoga is also about being joyful!

At the physical level, chanting *Om* helps in the control of the breath. It regulates the out-breath, lengthening it so that exhalation is fuller and the maximum amount of stale air is expelled. It stimulates the lung cells, giving a better exchange of gases, improves the circulation and stimulates the ductless glands.

The vibrations created by sounding *Om* also affect the chakras, the centres of energy in the subtle body. *Om* can be likened to "the Word" mentioned in St. John's Gospel. There is an almost identical passage to it in the *Rig Veda*, composed many centuries earlier: "In the beginning was Brahman; second to Him was the Word which was with Him, the Word is Brahman."

The *Bhagavad Gita*, the *Srimad Bhagavatam* and Patanjali's *Yoga Sutra* all contain passages on the significance of *Om*. The *Upanishads* also teaches about its importance and various sections reflect upon its meaning. Indeed, every *Upanishad* begins with *Om*:

> *Om stands for the Supreme Reality.*
> *It is a symbol for what was,*
> *what is, and what shall be.*
> *Om represents also what lies beyond past,*
> *present and future.*
> MANDUKYA UPANISHAD

Hari Om Tat Sat

Om is frequently used at the beginning of a mantra, such as the popular Tibetan *Om mani padme hum* mantra, which roughly translates as 'Homage to the jewel in the lotus'.

I was once asked to explain the expression *Hari Om Tat Sat*. Each one of these words is a name of the Divine Lord. So every time we repeat one of these words, we are chanting a name for God.

Traditionally a session of yoga practice begins and ends with *Om* or *Hari Om*. This reminds us of the true meaning and aim of yoga – to unite the whole of our being with the Divine. This is why many yoga students use *Om*, or *Hari Om*, at the beginning and end of any spiritual work or exercises.

The word *Tat* is used to renounce any reward, and *Sat* is the end of the work and practices that have been done. *Sat* is derived from the word *Satya*, which means 'truth'. Therefore, if it is God's work we are doing and it is offered to God – *Tat* – it is done in truth. Study the *Bhagavad Gita*, chapter 14, verses 23-28 and you will find it there. Some translations have quite a long commentary on this.

10

Our Limitless Inheritance

SANTOSHAN

Yoga is nothing but practical psychology.
SRI AUROBINDO

The greatest wisdom of yoga lies in a variety of techniques for discovering and understanding ourselves, and our authentic and limitless nature. An early synthesis of yoga philosophy and practice is Patanjali's *Yoga Sutra,* written around the 2nd century CE, although much of what is described in it can be traced back even further.

The *Sutra* teaches various concepts about the mind, ego and ways to the true Self that are crucial facets of yogic development. Patanjali's summary of ethical conduct, along with the *Sutra's* teachings on inner discipline, are important principles in many branches of yoga. Because of the essential teachings that the *Sutra* covers, the following pages includes some of them in order to outline key points about yogic spirituality, along with comparative Buddhist beliefs and other important perspectives.

Realising what has been forever drawing us to Its heart
The Sanskrit word *chitta* refers to the mind and consciousness. It can be employed to describe any mental process or internal state, such as recollection, memory, intuitive wisdom, our individual sense of self, the unconscious or lower functions of the mind and perception. Normally, we identify with our individual personalities; not realising there is a richer life to which we can awaken. Yoga teaches us about blindness of our true Selves, which causes self-centredness and separates us from the vast ocean of existence within and around us.

For many of the yogic seers, knowledge of our true Self and its implications is fully realised in deep states of meditation. Ordinary consciousness is transformed and transcended through various practices into superconscious awareness that realises a supreme state of Oneness with everything in the universe and beyond.

Pathways to the true Self

Like other great wisdom traditions, yoga views egoism and desires as prime causes of suffering. The overcoming of their negative influence is therefore important. Yet it is not about eradicating *all* desires, but more of a loosening up of wanting things to go our own way. Because of this, the cultivation of calmness and patience is particularly important – though the latter is not mentioned in the *Yoga Sutra* – along with awareness and mindfulness of what we are doing in the present moment.

Other practices are invariably a practical combination of individual development, meditation exercises, personal effort and responsibility and the nurturing of a flexible non-attachment – performed as a way to freedom and spontaneity in life, and to this end used in the quest to overcome inhibiting states of mind and binding actions.

It is essential to understand that non-attachment is not about being aloof and separate from life – just as we would not consider the cure of an illness as being about taking medicine that merely numbs our feelings and physical senses and makes us unaware of any pain. Non-attachment encompasses acknowledgment of and being unbound by any restrictive feeling or mental state.

There are various paths of development that are recommended, such as the path of devotion to the Divine, the path of selfless work, and the path of spiritual insight and wisdom. There are no clear boundaries between these, as they can each include aspects of one another when we perform them.

Patanjali's path, which is often termed Royal Yoga, lies in the application of various meditative states and in awakening to the true Self. It is also called 'psychological yoga' because of its emphasis on gaining power over the mind and emotions, and on learning how to focus one's awareness.

As in early Buddhism, Hindu Tantra and Sri Aurobindo's Integral

Yoga, Patanjali does not view life as an illusion. He sees suffering and unsatisfactoriness as part of the human condition and motivating the seeker to search for answers and solutions to life's problems. All things are seen to have a level of truth about them. After all, if we were to try walking through a mountain, would we not hurt ourselves?

Karma and introspection

We should not be inhibited by our conditioned existence, but seek to become disentangled from it in order to discover the authentic spiritual centre of our being. But this does not imply non-creative participation in life until we have become fully enlightened, as there are numerous practices within yoga which can be applied from the start, and will help us to become more spiritually aware and responsible forces for good in the world. It is in many ways seen as a gradually expanding and growing process towards discovering our authentic selves, which allows for spiritual living every step of the way.

Introspection into our deeper selves is advocated in order to become aware of any imprints or impressions which have formed within us, such as restrictive negative thoughts, feelings, impulses or actions. These impressions are termed *samskaras*, which form deep rooted patterns or traits (*vasanas*) that can affect our current and future states of being. Yet we can rise above these inhibiting patterns, as they do not absolutely determine our actions, because only the present moment exists and how we act in each moment is a matter of personal responsibility and free will. This obviously links us with ideas about karma and practices of mindfulness and awareness in both Buddhist and Hindu spirituality, and with exercises involving the creative use of the will.

The word karma literally means 'action' and refers to actions having consequences. How one produces skilful or unskilful karma and overcomes its binding influence can be interpreted differently by different traditions, or include a combination of different elements, such as whether a person fulfils his or her assigned duties, takes steps to avoid harming others, or is devoted to God.

In Buddhism and the early *Upanishads*, unskilful karmic actions are linked with desires. But it within Buddhism that I feel we get more fleshed-out practical teachings on it and explanations of how it is bound up with the intentions behind our actions. Additionally, purity, desires and ignorance – aspects of the *gunas*, which I will describe in more detail towards the end of this chapter – are three principal states of mind that are seen to create either beneficial or inhibiting *samskaras*. As in all the great wisdom traditions, purity of mind and heart are fundamental qualities to cultivate in yoga.

In the early Buddhist commentaries there is a list of what I see as five sensible categories of natural laws that are able to influence our lives, of which karma is linked with only *one* of them (the fourth category). These are:

(1) Physical objects and changes in the environment.
(2) Heredity.
(3) The workings of the mind.
(4) Human behaviour.
(5) The interrelationship and interdependence of all things.

Further to these, there are also the laws of society, which tie in with human thought and conduct and, therefore, also link up with ideas about karma. We can see from these laws that not everything that happens to us is necessarily to do with some past karmic action or influence being played out. A tree might be blown down and knock us on the head through no fault of our own; other than being in the wrong place at the wrong time. Or we might inherit genes from our parents that create a weakness in a particular area, or suffer the consequences of someone *else's* actions and carelessness. I think it also worth mentioning the insights Carl Jung had about the collective unconscious, which suggests there are other factors at play in the universe that need considering, before coming to conclusions about individual karmic influences in our life. Viewed psychologically, karma is nothing mysterious, but basic common sense about how unhealthy states of mind cause us to suffer.

The wisdom of insight
By cultivating insight into different states of mind we learn about ourselves and unskilful patterns created by our past actions, and

experiences and other influences that can affect us. With this comes the wisdom of knowing how to overcome barriers to spiritual living. For all our experiences and actions (emotional, mental, physical, spiritual) will leave subliminal imprints or impressions, which will influence us in either a positive or negative way – though sometimes the effect can be neutral.

If we are not careful, we can become entrapped in never-ending cycles of unskilful actions, where negative imprints and impressions continually affect our conscious state, which in turn creates further binding imprints and impressions that unwholesomely influence us even more:

> *Each thought, each feeling, each action of ours has a corresponding effect upon our consciousness, and consequently upon our life and nature.... But there is another complementary truth which has also to be borne in mind, that it is our consciousness that determines our thought, feeling and action.*
> RISHABHCHAND

These days we may think more in terms of the unconscious mind storing *samskaras*. The word *chitta* is sometimes used as a comparative because of its association with recollection and memory. But it was not until the 4th century CE that a more specific term was used in the Yogacara School of Buddhism, when the concept of *alaya-vijnana* was developed by its founder Asanga. It literally means 'store-consciousness' and is used to describe a subliminal reservoir of tendencies, habits, and future possibilities based on impressions of past experience and karmic actions, which subsequently influence all present and future modes of experience.

It could perhaps be argued that such a form of consciousness must have been something that was already there and understood in yoga practices, but that it had never been called a store-consciousness before – similar to how some modern psychologists and writers have given new labels to things that they did not have before.

Moving beyond the dance of restriction

Because of the influence of the *samskaras*, it is essential to use the introspective mind to become aware of any harmful or restrictive traits. Mantras and *pranayama* practices are particularly powerful methods for transforming negatives, such as low self-worth or feelings of guilt, as they help us to focus on more positive qualities within ourselves and on the creative force of life that flows through everything and everyone.

Higher uses of the will, reasoning and reflective abilities also help us to become more empowered, self-aware and wiser individuals. If we truly wish to live a spiritual life, we need to understand, accept and work on all levels – the good, moderate and imperfect – for the purpose of opening up the way to freedom and overcoming any limiting traits and their influence.

For some yoga students this implies not only working on psychological problems developed in this life, but also on any that have been produced in previous ones. It also means embracing the good within us. The teachings are not about original sin (which even Christian writers, such as Matthew Fox, have shown to have no place in either the teachings of Jesus or in those of numerous important Christian mystics), but realising unafflicted pure being and transforming anything that stops us from reflecting our more authentic Self that unites us with everything and everyone.

Strongly rooted negative impressions are a particular obstacle, as they continuously feed the mind with a stream of inhibiting activity. This is a psychological heritage we all have to work with. The impressions may be the product of our own actions, or caused by subliminal influences, and various factors of modern living and the pressure to fit in with a growing materialistic world that wants to make us dance its tune. Seeking the right kind of influences in one's life is therefore highly recommended. Yoga teaches that all inhibiting influences and aspects of ourselves can not only be known, but also conquered. Through the right application of the practices and exercises, all obstacles may be overcome.

Awakening to the One Life

The quest for enlightenment has always been a bit of a tricky process. On the one hand, it can lead us to becoming more spiritually whole and responsible. On the other, we may find ourselves using it as way of avoiding necessary work on the emotional and psychological levels of ourselves. John Welwood coined the phrase 'spiritual bypassing' to describe this. Even the most advanced masters and students can still exhibit problems connected with their individual psychological nature.

The safest approach to the growth of our complete personality needs to embrace not only a vertical process of transcendence, and an embodiment of higher levels and realisations, but also a horizontal process of including, harmonising and transforming the relative psychological parts of our being into a spiritual whole. It is a road that leads us to healthily transform anything that stops us from reflecting the spiritual essence of our being in all areas.

Questions about whether yoga was originally a path of escape from life or a path to wholeness and integration is quite an old one. The truth is that it has at times been used for both. It all comes down to where the emphasis is placed, how the teachings are interpreted and what practices are advocated. Obviously selfless service (karma yoga) and social commitments (*svadharma*) are about healthily engaging with everyday life, whereas becoming a recluse is the opposite of these. On the whole, the latter is rarely practised in the Hindu tradition. Krishna in the *Bhagavad Gita* encouraged Ajuna to fulfil his princely duties, instead of renouncing them in favour of an ascetic way of life. Marpa, the renowned Tibetan Buddhist yogi and one of the main gurus of the Kagyu lineage, was a farmer with a wife and seven children. As well as giving yogic instruction to students, he also had to oversee the work of labourers on his farm.

If our emphasis is solely on transcendence and the realisation of Ultimate Truths without looking at other realms of development and practical ways of living, then we are in danger of using spiritual exercises as a method of avoidance. In many ways the spiritual journey is about "aestheticism not asceticism", which as Matthew Fox reminds us, is about the art of living – living our life skilfully as a form spiritual practice – finding unity in diversity, and discovering and manifesting creative beauty in our development.

Looking at the life of the Buddha, we can see how he took a balanced middle path between complete renunciation and being fully involved in worldly life. Like the Zen Ox-herding pictures, where the seeker brings blessings to and takes part in ordinary life after enlightenment, the Buddha did not run away from everyday existence and frequently gave advice on how people could wholesomely conduct themselves in regular affairs.

Engagement in the world

Puzzlingly, Patanjali's interpretation of the final stage of enlightenment is generally seen as a state of isolation, inactivity and disinterest in the world. If it were not for the mention of everyday ethics in his teachings, we might mistakenly think he was advocating a path of no interest in worldly life. We have to remember that his *Yoga Sutra* is only a brief summary of teachings that had been around for some time. Other branches of yoga that incorporate the practices have come to different conclusions about enlightenment. Yet, for Patanjali the world is real and the Truth lies behind it. We could perhaps argue that once this Truth is realised we must surely recognise it as existing in everything and everyone and therefore implying that all life is part of this Reality.

In the book *The Integrity of the Yoga Darsana*, the writer Ian Whicher puts forward an excellent case for Patanjali's teachings being about the integration of all parts of ourselves – the moral, physical, emotional, mental and spiritual. This approach ties in with other wisdom traditions that are life affirming and is the central message of many contemporary teachers, who seek to encourage their students to find an active balance between spiritual engagement and healthy non-attachment within the world. It means rising above our everyday entanglements, and combining discernment with emotional and social responsibility; thus allowing us to participate in and respect life with spiritual understanding and display compassionate empathy towards others – awareness of our actions and reverence for the sacredness of life is highly prized in yogic wisdom.

The three *guna* qualities

Unique to the Hindu yogic tradition is the idea of the three *gunas*, described as qualities or components. They are seen as subtle substances and are believed to play an essential role in the way they interact with nature (*prakrti*) and to be the primary active components of

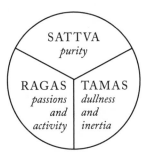

FIGURE 7: *The Three Gunas.*

all mental and physical material in the universe. In yogic texts they are individually described as 'purity' (*sattva*), 'activity, passions and desires' (*ragas*), and 'inertia and dullness' (*tamas*, connected also with ignorance).

Traditionally they have represented three different influential qualities, which react with and seek to dominate each other, and are seen as energies behind all psychological states of mind. Modern interpretations view *sattva guna's* energy as a harmonising force that balances the other two *gunas* and brings about a state of equanimity. This modern interpretation is not about being in just a *sattvic* state all the time, but, nonetheless, *sattva* is seen to be predominant in spiritual practices of mindfulness, generosity and compassion, as well as in intellectual, creative and virtuous thoughts and displays of self-mastery.

Ragas guna is looked upon as the energy behind all physical actions and desires, and playing a particularly important role in the creation of the universe. An unhealthy predominance of *tamas guna* is believed to produce narrow beliefs and lethargy, and is seen to be influential in times of inactivity. But it ought to be mentioned that there are higher and lower aspects to all three *gunas*.

If we analyse ourselves and observe life around us, we may notice what is seen to be the *gunas'* influence and energy at different times of the day. At night, for instance, we might observe the influence of *tamas* becoming more predominant as our minds become sluggish and restful. *Ragas*, on the other hand, is more noticeable during an active day. The following are further examples given in James Fadiman's and Robert Frager's excellent, *Personality and Personal Growth*:

In the process of creating a statue, for example, tamas can be seen in the untouched, inert stone. Ragas is the act of carving, and sattva is the image in the sculptor's imagination....

... Rich or heavy foods are tamasic because they are difficult to digest and cause laziness or sleepiness. Spicy hot foods are rajasic as they lead to activity, strong emotions, or nervousness. Fresh fruit and vegetables are sattvic and promote calmness. Certain places, such as mountains and the ocean shores are sattvic and thus suitable for spiritual practice.

When there is disharmony between the three *gunas*, it causes the mind to become imbalanced. This imbalance is seen by yogis to create a state of unenlightenment and a belief that material objects and worldly experience can give us lasting happiness. It is also seen to be responsible for creating the limited sense of self or 'I' which separates us from our real nature. Nonetheless, it is through the mind, with its higher functions of will, insight, intuition and wisdom (higher aspects of *buddhi*), that liberation from restrictive 'seer' and 'seen' worldly experience can be reached. Through the use of the will, true insight and pure *sattvic* knowledge we start to overcome our limitations and focus our attention on authentic levels of being.

Once we have done this, we then have to make the final leap of awakening to the difference between *sattvic* knowledge and our Ultimate Nature. Yogic texts tell us that at this stage we will then no longer be under the *gunas'* influence or inhibited by physical existence – we will awaken to unbound freedom, and unity with all life and the Supreme Divine Self will arise naturally within us.

Anatomy of evolution and individualised being

Understanding our psychic and physical being as constituting a symbolic miniature of the creative elements in the cosmos, is a common theme in yogic belief and part of its alchemy to Self-realisation. *Figure 8* is a basic diagram of different aspects of ourselves, based on Samkhya yoga's model, which is frequently found with minor adjustments and additions in different schools and teachings of yoga. *Purusha* is looked upon as the transcendental pure Self in Samkhya Yoga. In various

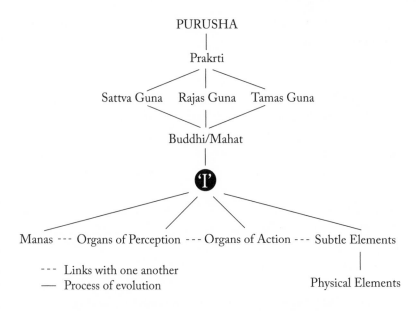

FIGURE 8: *Samkhya Philosophy's Model of Evolution and the Whole Self.*

Purusha: the transcendental pure Self in Samkhya. In other yogic traditions it is the witness conscious, the individual spirit and seen as either a projection of, or identical with, the *atman*.

Prakrti: unmanifest, primal nature – connected with the Creative Goddess energy (Shakti) in Tantra yoga.

Sattva Guna: pureness and equilibrium.

Rajas Guna: activity, passions and desires.

Tamas Guna: inertia, dullness and ignorance.

Buddhi: intuitive and discriminating faculty (higher and lower intellect and the manifestation of wisdom) and linked with the individual conscious will.

Mahat: cosmic intelligence that arose at the beginning of Creation.

'I': the *ahamkara* – individual sense of self – the ego.

Manas: the lower mind through which we receive impressions – the processing of sensory information.

Organs of Perception: ear, skin, eye, tongue and nose.

Organs of Action: voice, hand, feet, procreation and excretion.

Subtle Elements: the five *tanmatras* – sound, touch, sight, taste and smell.

Physical Elements: the five *mahabhutas* – space/ether, air, fire, water and earth.

yogic traditions it is also seen as the higher witness consciousness, the individual conscious spirit personality or soul, and is viewed as either a projection of, or identical with, the *atman*.

The components of the diagram are viewed not only as a psychological representation of ourselves, but also as a metaphysical model for how the universe and human life came into being. *Mahat* is the level of Cosmic Intelligence. The role of the 'I' or *ahamkara* (the I-maker) is seen to play a part in producing non-material blueprints for sound, touch, sight, taste and smell, as well as providing the potential for basic individual abilities. The idea of the universe being created by the sacred sound and vibration of *Om* happens at the subtle elements (*tanmatras*) level.

In the *Yoga Sutra*, the mind consists of three components: *manas*, *buddhi* and the 'I'. In the philosopher Shankara's system, space, air, fire, water and earth are subtle elements which first produce sound, touch, sight, taste and smell, followed by the equivalent physical elements. Shankara also added the chief breath of life (*muhyaprana*) which divides into five energies (*pranas*), subserving different functions of respiration and the body. Awakening to the power and purified use of *paranic* energy is an essential in almost all yogic schools.

Devotional schools include a personal God, with whom students seek to either accomplish union with or recognise that they are an intrinsic part of, and link *prakrti* with the Creative Mother Goddess (Shakti). In Tantra yoga, neither the male (Shiva) nor female (Shakti) forms of the Divine are seen as either superior or inferior to one another and are invariably viewed as expressions of a formless Supreme Reality:

> *Within Shiva there is Shakti, within Shakti there is Shiva. I see no*
> *difference between them; they are like the moon and the moonlight.*
> Siddhasiddhanta Sangraha

11

The Divine with a Feminine Face

SWAMI DARMANANDA

The Goddess in all her manifestations [is] ...
a symbol of the unity of all life in Nature.
MARIJA GIMBUTAS

Much is often written about the Divine in Its absolute form (Nirguna Brahman). Yoga and Tantra invariably tell us about Shiva and Shakti, the passive masculine and the active creative feminine energy. These can be viewed as abstract ways of understanding and experiencing something of the Divine working in nature, and beyond our individual selves and the universe. The Divine Feminine is traditionally linked with creativity and the Earth in just about all spiritual traditions. Because of this I felt impelled to write something about Saraswati, one of the popular Goddess figures, to give a balanced view of the richness of the Hindu and yogic tradition.

It can be said that if we did not approach the Divine in a personalised way it would be difficult to comprehend anything about Divinity and the sacredness of life within and around us. We often need to approach the Divine in an individual way before opening to wider knowledge and understanding. The various Gods and Goddesses of India all represent One Ultimate Reality. The Hindu spiritual tradition is not polytheistic, as sometimes believed, but generally either monotheistic or monistic, depending on the teachings followed.

The personalised forms found in temples and devotees' homes help people to understand something about the Divine and Its abundant qualities (Saguna Brahman), such as love and forgiveness, as well as something about its Ultimate Transcendence. They remind devotees of their relationship with the Divine, the spiritual qualities within them, and the Divine as everyone's individualised being and consciousness.

In the West we have, rightly or wrongly, tended to focus on posture work, the practices of meditation and on intellectual philosophies of yoga, and often overlook the important symbolism depicted in various statues and paintings, and how they can help us to focus our minds on higher aspects of ourselves and realise our profound unity with all life upon the Earth.

Goddess worship is Hinduism at its more popular level. She is often found, in one aspect or another, as the main deity of many small villages in India. The following pages of this chapter are a description of the Goddess Saraswati and what she profoundly represents.

The Divine Mother Saraswati

The *Mahabharata* says, "Behold Saraswati, Mother of the *Vedas* abiding in me". The Divine Mother is everywhere and manifests in many forms. Saraswati is revered in both Tibetan Buddhism, and in the Hindu spiritual tradition, and was extremely popular in the medieval period of Nepal.

In one of her aspects, she is Brahma-Shakti, seen in conjunction with the personalised Hindu God Brahma and considered to be his consort. She is also seen as the knowledge behind the power of Brahman, the Supreme Absolute, and the Devi of speech, art, music and wisdom.

Ramachandra said that Saraswati is a "Goddess full of *knowledge* and flowing stream of *wisdom*, divine speech inspired from *Ritam*, truth, consciousness, inner illumination and insight, enlightening all undertakings". It is said that she resides in all the chakras as the Devi of speech. Her seed mantra is '*Aim*', which can be interpreted in the following way:

Ai = Saraswati
m = Bindu (the dispeller of sorrow)

We, through the worship of Saraswati – or what she signifies – gain the bounty to speak words of truth and inspiration to others, which helps to create harmony amongst those around us. One of the traditional prayers to Saraswati is the following one:

Oh Devi! O Saraswati!
Reside thou ever in my speech.
Reside thou ever on my tongue tip
O Divine Mother, giver of faultless poetry!

Saraswati is known as the Supreme Devi, Mother of the *Vedas* and of all worlds. The Goddess Saraswati is depicted clothed in white garments. Her vehicle is a swan, peacock or lotus flower. Her beautiful smiling face is always serene. Her hair is dark in colour and she is often shown with four arms depicting different aspects, qualities and powers of her nature. In two hands she holds a 'veena' (a stringed musical instrument). In another she holds a book or scroll. In a fourth hand she holds a *japa-mala* (beads used for counting repeated chants and mantras). In some cases she holds a lotus blossom (a type of water lily), a symbol of purity and of humankind's spiritual growth from the mud that lies at the bottom of ponds to a flower with its petals open to the pure rays of the sun.

In her headdress there is usually set the eye of a peacock's tail feather. Her smiling countenance and posture radiate harmony and peace. Her

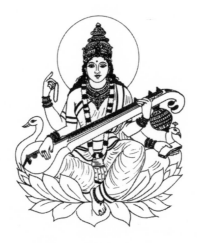

FIGURE 9: *The Goddess Saraswati.*

name denotes 'flow' or 'motion' (*saras*). Her smiling countenance shows compassion and benevolence to those who seek her bounty.

Her white garments represent the colour of *akasa* and *buddhi*, which are symbols of purity and uncontaminated wisdom. The veena is often regarded as the only instrument capable of producing pure melody. So we see that Saraswati has qualities of harmony and creativity, through sound vibrations depicted by this musical instrument. The veena also denotes all sounds (*sabda*) of which Saraswati is the Mother.

The book or scroll is seen as the wisdom of God and/or the ancient *Srimad Bhagavatam*, which is said to contain the teachings of the highest knowledge and wisdom. The *japa-mala* is a reminder of the importance of mantra (sound), including the creative vibrations of *Om* and *So-ham/Hamsa* (the latter being a variation of *So-ham* and a name also given to the saints who have attained God Consciousness), and the unbroken remembrance of God and truth.

Saraswati's vehicles

Her lotus vehicle – along with the fore-mentioned points about the flower – is a symbol of love and of the blossoming of higher consciousness, creation and evolution. The peacock feather represents the many-faceted glory of the Spirit. The eye in the peacock feather can also be seen to represent the all-seeing eyes of the Divine Mother, as well the insight of spiritual wisdom. It can also symbolise the third eye or even vanity that has to be overcome in order to reach a true state of enlightenment.

The swan which accompanies her, or on which she is sometimes depicted riding, is also a symbol of wisdom. The swan is said to have the ability to separate milk from water when the two have been mixed, so reminding us that wisdom consists in the ability of being able to discern spiritual truth and knowledge from watered-down and unnecessary rituals or dogmas, or from unclear teachings.

Sir John Woodroffe pointed out that in Tantric texts the swan is *Ham-sa*, which is no material bird, but a symbol for the vital force (*pranic* energy) manifesting as the inhaling *Sa/So* and the exhaling *Ham* breath. This universal force acts within all life.

We see from these symbols how Saraswati is regarded as the

Goddess of life, wisdom, learning and intelligence, and is the patron of students, scholars and artists. To use Sir John Woodroffe's words, "She ... is the Divine in the aspect as Wisdom and learning, for she is the Mother of Veda, that is, of all knowledge touching Brahman and the Universe ... not therefore idly have men worshipped *Vak* or Saraswati as the Supreme Power". Swami Radha pointed out how she is also bound up with inspiration and the harmonious aspects of life:

> *Appreciation of the harmonious aspects of life is personified in Saraswati, the Goddess of speech, of art, of music. When we can speak words of inspiration that touch an inner chord in another person, we can say that this is the worship of the Goddess Saraswati. We thereby have created our own world of harmony in which we function.*
> SWAMI RADHA

A *Vedic* hymn to Saraswati pleads with her to open her "beautiful form containing the treasures of Vedic wisdom, for us to behold and drink deep the soma juice of exhilarating delight". Saraswati also has associations with the main *nadis* (energy channels in the subtle body). In Tantric texts it describes that, "In the *Ida* is the Devi Yamuna and in *Pingala* is Saraswati and in *Susumna* dwells Ganga". There is a variation of this shown in the *Sammahana Tantra*, which reads, "In the *Ida* is the Devi Jahnavi and Yamuna is in *Pingala*, and Saraswati is in *Susumna*".

These names also refer to three sacred rivers, which were said to have joined at Allahabad, just as the three *nadis* (energy channels) are said to conjoin at the three *granthis* (meaning 'knots'). This shows the conjunction of the three rivers with the Saraswati River in the centre, which is believed to have disappeared thousands of years ago. But, of course, the Ganges is perhaps the best known river in India and the Jumna River still flows into the Ganges. Interestingly, in 1988 an article appeared in a daily newspaper describing the discovery underground of the Saraswati River while engineers were drilling for oil in the hills and valleys of the Shivaliks, near Dehra Dun.

Saraswati and mantra

There are certain days which are associated with particular deities.

If one wishes to take advantage of a particular auspicious day, then a mantra for the appropriate deity should be chanted. If you already have a mantra, this is chanted first.

Auspicious days for Saraswati fall between mid-January and mid-February, five days after the new moon and between mid-September to mid-October. Seven to nine days after the new moon.

The mantra *Jaya Saraswati* can be chanted, or *Om Sri Saraswati Namali* (Hail to Saraswati), or *Mangalum dishtu me Saraswati* (May Saraswati give me auspiciousness). There are many others. Saraswati is also included in one of the numerous triplets represented by *Om*: the three Devis, Saraswati, Lakshmi and Durga. Each deity will reveal their truth and spiritual aspect behind their form to the sincere devotee.

May Saraswati, Divine Mother, shower her blessings upon you.

12
Steps to Authentic Being

SANTOSHAN

Patanjali's *Yoga Sutra* consists of a hundred and ninety-five short aphorisms, divided into four parts. Much remains unsaid, which is probably because some topics and practices were all too evident at the time and needed little explanation.

Within the *Sutra* are the essential eight-steps or limbs of yoga (*astanga* yoga). They outline a classical route taken by many students, from daily life practices to superconscious spiritual awakening. These steps have become central to various systems of yoga, and are looked upon as important stages that follow on from one another, beginning with the most practical and leading on to knowledge of one's pure, free and wise nature. They are not found in the philosopher Shankara's Advaita Vedanta system however, which can be seen as more of a top-down approach, which focuses more on the *atman*-Brahman relationship than on evolving stages that start with ethical behaviour. Modern integralism, on the other hand, might consider starting where one is strongest and expanding from that point to include the whole of one's being. Swami Nikhilananda also wrote about this being the approach of the *Bhagavad Gita* in his translation of the work.

The eight-steps themselves are looked upon as a process of mental and emotional purification, and includes practices found in other wisdom traditions, such as self-awareness, purifying the heart and bringing about positive changes in one's life and outlook.

Steps for spiritual unfoldment: the eightfold path of yoga
1. Ethical conduct (yamas)
Under the heading of *yamas*, which literally means 'restraints', but might be better understood as observations, are five ethical rules:

(1) Non-violence in thought, word and deed.
(2) Truthfulness.
(3) Non-stealing.
(4) Chastity.
(5) Greedlessness and non-grasping.

The five observations above are seen as different areas for spiritual development and ways of avoiding negative behaviour. Number 4 can be translated to mean moderation in all activities. We should consider the fact that some yoga teachers belong to family lineages that can be traced back several generations. They would, therefore, not be expected to observe the practice of celibacy all the time, otherwise their lineages would die out. The Buddhist precept of abstaining from sexual misconduct might be a more practical interpretation, as sex is not dismissed as something unsacred in the Hindu tradition. Bede Griffiths reminded us about this in his writings on the symbolism of the *Shiva-lingam*, and pointed out how it is invariably looked upon as holy and linked with the Supreme Creative Source of all:

> *The sexual origin of the* lingam *is, of course, obvious, but this only brings out the extraordinary depth of understanding of ancient India. Sex was always regarded as something 'holy' – I think it still is, except where the Indian spirit has been corrupted by the West. The* lingam *was therefore a natural symbol of the sacred 'source of life.'*

At no point are we told to follow the eightfold-path of yoga blindly, but we are meant to reflect upon how we can apply it and how far we need to go with it. The practice of discernment and taking responsibility for one's spiritual growth is highly valued in all the great wisdom traditions and needs be used by all students of spirituality when deciding what is helpful for their growth. We should not judge ourselves harshly if we feel we have not lived-up to some of the key principles of yoga, as we cannot achieve everything overnight and feelings of guilt are counterproductive to healthy development.

The eightfold path of yoga needs to be seen as a guide only for steering us on the right path. Like all spiritual teachings, we have to interpret them for ourselves, come to our own conclusions and decide how much is right for us. This is all part of the development process. There can be good reasons for acting less than we feel we should; often it is because we are suffering – mentally, physically or emotionally – or feel that our spiritual life is being overpowered by events beyond our control. The latter can be found underlying many of our feelings of discontentment.

A friend once told a Psychosynthesis group she was involved in how lucky she was, as she had lots of problems to work on in her development! It can be helpful to look at our life and growth with a similar understanding and realise that it is here that initial work is invariably done. We must ask ourselves whether there are any past issues affecting our current understanding and judgments about life and people. We also need to see whether our surroundings, work, friends and relationships are creative forces in our lives – consciously or unconsciously. If not, what can we do to make them more wholesome and supportive?

A good way of starting the five *yamas*/observations is to sit quietly for a while then write down one of them and think about what it means. See what thoughts or feelings arise. Think about how you can apply it and how you can overcome any barriers which are causing problems in your spiritual journey – it may be about letting go, working on past issues or towards a goal, or transforming something in the present. Ask yourself if you need to practise the *yama* all the time and whether there are times when it is not possible to apply it and why.

If you write down your thoughts, feelings and insights in a diary, it will help to make them more concrete, instead of being just passing impressions. It will also give you something to later reflect upon and see how you are progressing. Swamiji once pointed out that we do not have to think about applying all the *yamas*, but take just one of them and live by it. An example she gave for this was the practice of non-violence (*ahimsa*), which can be seen as the main principle of many great teachers, such as Jesus, Mahatma Gandhi and Martin Luther King Jr. and as being the most important *yama*.

2. Inner virtues and mastery (niyamas)

Whereas the *yamas* focus on ethical conduct, the *niyamas* are concerned with inner virtues and mastery and are intended to regulate one's relationship with the spiritual life. The five *niyamas* are:

(1) Inner purity, which includes the purifying of one's mind and loosening material attachments.

(2) Contentment (a state of equanimity, calmness and composure), which comes about through the practice of inner purity.

(3) Austerity, implying practices such as fasting, observing silence or stillness, in which the student removes impurities and establishes a greater power over his or her senses, but does not imply extreme asceticism.

(4) Self-study, which has a double meaning of contemplating scripture and various sciences, as well as of mindful introspection, self-acceptance and understanding.

(5) Devotion to the Lord (*ishvara*), which is defined in the *Yoga Bhasya* (an influential commentary on the *Sutra*) as the offering up of all actions to the Supreme Teacher, and which is comparable to the joint practice of devotion and karma yoga found in the *Bhagavad Gita*. One of the most famous practices of devotion is the recitation of *Om*: seen as a creative and an ever-present manifestation of the Divine in the universe.

3. Posture (asana)

The first two steps regulate our contact with everyday life and are intended to reduce unskilful acts which bind us to conditioned worldly existence (*samsara*: the world of change and unsatisfactoriness, which is linked also with rebirth). The overall aim is to eradicate all karma and inhibiting impressions. But to take the process a step further, we have to find the right place where we will not be interrupted and able to still our bodies by using a particular meditation posture, which will aid single-pointed concentration.

Obviously it is not possible for us all to rush off to the Himalayas and meditate in a nice quiet cave and this is not what Patanjali suggests doing. Nonetheless, we can either find a peaceful location, spiritual place or centre, or put aside a quiet area or room in our homes that we can use solely for the purpose of meditation practice.

Having the right environment and posture will help to bring about physical, mental and emotional stability and aids meditation exercises. The *Yoga Sutra* states that the posture should be steady and comfortable. If the posture is incorrect, it can cause distractions, such as trembling of the body, pain or erratic breathing, and should be corrected. To illustrate how a regular place of spiritual practice can build energy and a more conducive environment for meditation, I should mention a small and ancient Shiva temple that Glyn Edwards and I once visited, which some Indian friends said we should experience first-hand.

It took us several hours to travel to it from Mumbai, along a dusty and winding road, congested with colourfully painted lorries. The temple had been used as a place of worship for hundreds of years and is believed to be one of the oldest in India. It had been built in a sacred area, next to a holy mountain. Inside, the low ceiling and walls were blackened with age. Various bulky, square-cut columns and a tiny shrine area that stepped-down from the main hall, gave the impression of being inside a cave. Squatted in the only available space were several yogis absorbed in mantra practice. The minute we entered the temple structure we both experienced an overwhelming energy that seemed to come up from deep within the earth and vibrate throughout the whole building. Both of us had never experienced anything quite like it before.

Unfortunately – or fortunately, depending on how you look at it – it was a busy but special holy day. The temple's attendants were frantically shuffling in pilgrims in one entrance, past the main shrine area, then out of a back exit. It meant there was no space or time allowed to just sit and be quiet. We could only image how deep one would have gone in such a place, especially with the aid of that kind of energy and atmosphere.

4. Control of the life-force (pranayama)

When the *asana* is practised correctly it supports the internalisation of our awareness. The next step is about energising through the practice of *pranayama*, which is performed to increase internalised awareness and bring about changes within us.

Pranayama is not only to do with the breath and practices involving

125

its retention and expansion whilst holding different *mudras* and *bandhas* (hand and body positions/locks), but also bound-up with the all-pervading, rejuvenating energy and life-force of the cosmos. This energy is focused on and creatively used in yogic spirituality (see Swamiji's *Life Energy* chapter for more details).

Patanjali's *Sutra* first mentions making the respiratory system as slow and steady as possible – obviously without force. Mircea Eliade pointed out that the practice of concentrating on the rhythm of the breath could well go back to early ritual chanting. The benefits of using the breath for relaxation and meditation purposes are almost endless. When our breathing is calm, regulated and rhythmic our minds, bodies and emotions become more peaceful. "The first sign of an uncontrolled mind", Swami Adiswarananda reminds us, "is irregularity of breathing".

5. Withdrawing the mind from the world of emotional and sensory distractions (pratyahara)

For most people, sitting quietly will still mean being distracted by various random thoughts, feelings and physical sensations. For this reason, the next step is about disidentifying from any distractions.

The word *pratyahara* is used to describe this process and is invariably interpreted as 'sensual-withdrawal', which does not imply blocking sensory distractions. If we consider what happens when we become engrossed in a book or any absorbing activity, we see how our mind and senses may still register other things, but do not get distracted by them. *Pratyahara* is about taking a mental step-back. Even if our minds are drawn away from this practice, we can still return to it without any effort.

Through the withdrawal of our minds from any emotional or sensory distractions we start to cultivate deep inner awareness. This is seen to reduce attachments to external surroundings and as an important stage of yogic meditation. Some yoga teachers recommend doing preliminary visualisation practice, which can help in achieving *pratyahara*.

It is worth mentioning that the Christian Father, Swami Amaldas made observations about positive and negative approaches to the practice of *pratyahara* in his book *Christian Yogic Meditation*. The negative approach occurs when we see ourselves in disharmony with anything that distracts us, including our own senses. It's a good point which can indeed lead to developing a negative view of distractions. His answer to this possible problem is to be aware of the outside world first and then bring it to the centre of one's being, so that everything becomes a part of our practice:

> *the withdrawal in its deepest sense is not that I separate myself from other beings ...*
>
> *After this kind of Prathyahara when I open my eyes, when I come out of meditation, I will be able to relate myself to others. The love and concern for others will flow spontaneously. I will still have the consciousness that everything around me is part of me.*
> SWAMI AMALDAS

This practice has some similarities with the practice of *antar mouna* (described by Swamiji in chapter 5). Much as I love the thinking behind Swami Amaldas's approach, I wonder how easy it is to achieve for anyone living in a violent and noisy neighbourhood. *Prathyahara* in its traditional form is something that can happen quite naturally when we have mastered the art of sitting quietly and focusing on our breath. This practice of going deep within oneself, taking some time out and recharging one's batteries and disidentifying from the world of the senses is known for bringing about great benefits – spiritually, creatively, mentally and emotionally.

Perhaps the answer lies in our preconceptions and the overall aim of what we are trying to achieve in our meditation practices. For instance, if on the one hand we are aiming to escape from the world, then the preliminary practice of *prathyahara* might help us to do that. On the other hand, if we look upon practising it as a step towards helping us to become more balanced and in tune with life, then it may help us move towards that goal.

6. Focusing the mind (dharana)

Following on from *pratyahara* is the holding of the mind in a motionless state, which is often described as 'one-pointed awareness'.

Dharana comes from the root word *dhr* meaning 'to hold'. It means directing the mind towards a specific object and keeping it focused on that in order to develop what is described as meditative absorption.

The object of concentration can be a physical one. Or it can be on a thought, an internal area, such as the heart-centre or, with the aid of mantra, focused on God. The *Yoga Sutra* mentions various distractions and obstacles that can weaken our commitment to both focusing our mind and our spiritual practices, such as ill-health, tiredness, being too worldly and doubt. Though I must admit to having seen a healthy element of doubt leading people to question things more deeply in their lives and development, and to become more mature, inclusive and less narrow in their spiritual beliefs.

The *Sutra*, like other teachings of yoga, encourages us to be vigilant and persevere in order to overcome any distractions and recommends one-pointed awareness as the best method for keeping them at bay. Other practices mentioned for overcoming obstacles and aiding peaceful states of mind and concentration, are the cultivation of positive qualities, including taking joy in other people's successes, equanimity and developing compassion and friendliness towards others. These are identical to Buddhism's four sublime states. There is also mention of the Buddhist practice of cultivating opposite thoughts to any distractions or negative states of mind.

A simple and popular practice for focusing the mind on an object (though not mentioned in the *Sutra*) is to place a lighted candle approximately 3 feet away from you, where you can gaze gently upon it. Look softly at the flame for a few minutes and notice all you can about it, i.e. its colour, brightness and the aura glowing around it. Then close your eyes and see if you can hold the image of the flame within your mind's eye (just above the middle of the eyebrows). After a few minutes, open your eyes and repeat the practice a few more times, then sit quietly for a while.

In the remaining steps of yoga's eightfold path you will see how this practice naturally flows into them.

7. Meditative absorption (dhyana)

Meditative absorption (*dhyana*) is a deeper stage that comes after focusing the mind, where the object concentrated upon becomes more tangible and vivid and *starts* to fill one's consciousness without distraction. It is seen to quieten and overcome various mental activities, states of mind and unconscious influences, such as a lack of knowledge of one's authentic Self, strong attachments to pleasures and aversions to anything one finds unpleasant. These gradually diminish as the meditative state expands and becomes more stable. Deep superconscious awareness is realised when all inhibiting states and unconscious distractions are finally transcended.

Pratyahara, focusing the mind and meditative absorption are all steps in the same process of internalisation, which lead to the final stage of the eightfold path of yoga.

8. *Superconscious knowledge of our true Selves (samadhi)*

The *Yoga Sutra* distinguishes between two types of *samadhi*. The first covers all kinds of insights and serene states that can be experienced by focusing on an object for meditation purposes (*samprajnata-samadhi:* aided superconsciousness). This kind of practice requires prolonged and deep meditative absorption so that the object of meditation fills one's entire consciousness, and brings about a fusion between the mind and the object concentrated on. Once accomplished, tranquil experiences of peace and calm arise naturally within ourselves.

The second type of *samadhi* is achieved without the aid of any objects (*asamprajnata-samadhi:* objectless superconsciousness). When achieved it is seen as a more complete stage towards realising our Ultimate Self.

It should perhaps be pointed out that *samadhi* is not an unconscious trance state; there is no loss of lucidity. Rather a sense of wakefulness and clarity is intensified. The experience of unbound freedom happens when ordinary consciousness is quietened and all opposites are transcended. It is the realisation of the higher Self, and liberation from the influence and bondage of unhealthy conditioning and our lower nature (*apara-prakrti*), of which the latter is intrinsically bound-up with the *gunas*. For the devotional practitioner, it is at this stage that the revelation of the Lord (*ishvara*), the Supreme Self, is revealed.

Liberation is about becoming consciously aware of and overcoming our false identifications with the ego-centred self and fully realising our authentic nature, which is ever-pure, wise and free. It does not imply that we get transported to another place or attain something that we did not have before. Swami Adiswarananda gives us a wonderful description about it in his superb book *Meditation and Its Practices*:

> *It is the Self-Realization – a burning realization that destroys all that is false and imaginary in us and reveals before us our true Self. Psychologically, it is rousing ourselves from self-centred inner polarization, division, and distraction to experience the reality of unified and harmonious existence.*

The states of *samadhi* are often described as blissful and are stages towards the final work of transforming and transcending all limiting aspects of ourselves. This includes the higher levels of reasoning and intuition (*buddhi*) and even *sattvic* knowledge (influence of the purity *guna*); although all these are valid, worked on and used in the process towards yogic enlightenment. In yogic thought, even in its purest form, *buddhi* is still considered to be under the influence of the *gunas* and believed to play a part in the creation of the separate ego-self. As long as there is a distinction between seer and seen reality we will not discover a complete awakening to the sacred Oneness of all. For even in the highest insights and greatest leaps of intuition there can still be traces of this distinction.

Perhaps the way to look at this is to think of higher functions and aspects of *buddhi* and *sattvic* knowledge as qualities of, or reflecting, the authentic spiritual Self, but not as the Ultimate in Its purest sense. Therefore, they also have to be transcended. Most yogic texts make this point, including the *Uddhava Gita*:

> *With mind thus calmed, overcome even sattva*
> *through continued dispassion towards the material world.*
> *Thus the wise overcome all three gunas,*
> *release themselves from the idea of 'I',*
> *and fix their attention on the absolute Self.*

13
Creative Life Energy

SWAMI DARMANANDA

Life is breath and breath is life.
So long as there is breath in the body there is life.
So to prana we should sing all hymns of praise.
Prana is the essence of the life breath.
And what is the life breath? It is pure consciousness.
And what is pure consciousness? It is the life breath.

KAUSHITAKI UPANISHAD

As we know breath is life. It is the first and last thing we do in this life. Various *pranayama* exercises improve the introduction of oxygen into the physical body and the removal of carbon dioxide. This in itself brings about good physiological benefits. But *pranayama* actually utilises the breathing process as a means to manipulate all forms of *prana* (life energy) within the human framework, whether gross or subtle.

In Swami Sivananda's informative book on the subject (*Science of Yoga: Vol. 7*) he points out that, "Pranayama is the control of the prana, and the vital forces of the body". This in turn has repercussions on the mind and physical body.

Defining *prana*
So often *pranayama* is introduced as breathing exercises or breath control. Possibly through translation difficulties. Compared with the English alphabet, Sanskrit has nearly twice as many letters with more than three times the number of vowels. Therefore, a large number of Sanskrit characters have no English equivalent. It is usually said that the words *prana* (breath) and *yama* (control) give us the word

131

pranayama, and therefore means 'breath control' or 'control of *prana*'.

However, some authorities say the actual word is not *yama,* but *ayama,* giving us *prana* plus *ayama: prana-ayama. Ayama* is defined as restraining, stretching, extending and expanding (implying the expansion of dimensions in time and space); thus *pranayama* means to extend and overcome one's normal limitations. The practice provides a method through which we can attain awareness of higher states of vibratory energy. In other words, we are able to regulate the *prana* comprising our human framework, and thereby make ourselves more sensitive to vibrations within and beyond us.

Pranayama is a method of refining the make-up of one's *pranic* body, one's physical body and also one's mind. By the correct practise of *pranayama* one's mind becomes calm and still, through which pure consciousness is then allowed to shine through without distortion.

The practice of *pranayama* brings new levels of awareness by quietening, stopping or restraining distractions of the mind. This restraint of mental activities allows us to know the higher levels of existence; like cleaning dirty windows to allow the sun to beam through, and to help us see it in its true glory.

The theory of *prana*

If we are to practise *pranayama*, it is helpful to examine the nature of *prana*. Swami Sivananda also tells us that, "*Prana* is the sum total of all energy that is manifest in the universe". In yoga the whole of the cosmos is said to be composed of two materials:

Prana – primal energy (or just energy)
Akasa – primordial nature (ether)

We can link these in with Shakti and *prakrti* as Santoshan has done in the *Where Everything Interconnects* chapter. Some yogic teachings don't mention Shakti at all and only talk about *pranic* energy. In these teachings *prana* is seen as a supreme energy acting in the universe, instead of it being a form of Shakti. It depends on whether the teaching is an early or later development in yogic history and if it is sympathetic towards, or has been influenced by, elements of

Tantra or Kundalini yoga.

Everything that possesses form or has material existence evolved out of *akasa*. Air, liquids, solid forms, the solar system, or any other such system in the universe, which may be said to be 'created', are products of the subtle *akasa*. When *akasa* takes physical form it becomes perceptible to us through the physical senses. At the end of its cycle as a material substance, it melts back into a formless subtle substance again. Therefore, the cycle from and to *akasa* is a perpetual one.

Every form of energy, such as the force of motion, light, heat, electricity, thought, etc., is derived from *prana*. All forces come out of *prana* and at the end of their cycle dissolve back into it.

At this point it may be appropriate to consider the laws of physics, which tell us that energy can be transformed but never destroyed. For example, electricity can be transformed into heat and light – as witnessed in our homes when we switch on electricity to obtain these. Chemicals, for example coal, can be transformed into electrical energy and so on. Readers will no doubt think of other examples.

Prana may be defined as the finest vital force in everything that is perceptible: on the physical plane as motion and action and on the mental plane as thought. It is the very essence of cosmic life – a subtle principle which evolved the whole universe into its present form, and is seen to be pushing it towards its ultimate goal.

When we begin to understand that *prana* is more than a personal principle, we realise that through the practice of *pranayama* our individual energy and consciousness can be expanded into universal energy and consciousness. If we consider that *prana* is linked with all activity in the cosmos, and that all our physical and mental actions have a co-relationship with this cosmic activity, it must then follow that our actions can have both a personal and universal effect. Just as the action of every cell of our body has an individual effect upon us, and likewise we are each a cell of the Universal Body which connects all life.

Five vital forces
We have seen how it can be said that *pranayama* means the control,

expansion and extension of universal *prana*. According to yogic texts, *prana* is divided into five main groups and five sub-groups. Let us look at the main groups first:

Prana:	The force which carries the breath inside.
Apana:	The force enabling the expelling of breath.
Udana:	The force by which we are able to act, due to the strength of the muscles.
Samana:	The force which maintains balance and co-ordination between all vitalities.
Vyana:	The force situated in the navel, the centre responsible for the metabolism and digestive system.

Pranayama is the extension of these forces and enables us to gain control over these functions. Through certain breathing exercises and techniques, purification of the nerves (the *nadis*) in the subtle anatomy comes about. A passage in the *Srimad Bhagavatam* reminds of this and tells us to, "Practise *pranayama* for the purification of the nerves". It is only then that *pranayama* is truly seen to begin.

The uniting of two of the principal *pranas* (*prana* and *apana*) is a fundamental aim: taking the united *prana* and *apana* slowly upwards towards the crown of the head. The practice of *pranayama* is an act of purification and a prerequisite to the practice of meditation.

The five sub-groups of *prana* are:

Naga:	Responsible for belching and hiccuping.
Koorma:	Opens the eyes.
Krikara:	Includes hunger and thirst.
Devadatta:	Responsible for yawning.
Dhananjaya:	Responsible for decomposition of the body after death.

Applications of *pranayama*

It is said that yoga is, "the stilling of the thought-waves of the mind" (*Yoga Sutra*). *Pranayama* is considered to help us towards this goal. When the breath is flowing harmoniously, then the fluctuations of the mind begin to still and bring about inner peace and balance:

And when the body is in silent steadiness, breathe rhythmically through the nostrils with peaceful ebbing and flowing of the breath. The chariot of the mind is drawn by wild horses, and these wild horses have to be tamed.
SVETASVATARA UPANISHAD

The fruit of *pranayama* is in an awakening to our higher spiritual consciousness. The first step towards this goal must surely be breath awareness. We know that we breathe, but are we aware of the breath? If we practise breath awareness with yoga postures, we can gradually extend our breath, utilising all of the lung area. Also the tone of the intercostal muscles can be improved.

Let us remember that just as we would approach yoga postures with care and discretion, so we should engage in *pranayama* exercises with the same attitudes. It ought to be mentioned that in some of the yogic text *pranayama* is performed *after* posture work, as suggested by the sequence of the eight-limbs in Patanjali's *Yoga Sutra*. Posture work itself, although done with breath work, prepares the way for pure *pranayama* practices – except it can be argued that sitting while doing *pranayama* is practising it with a posture.

In the *Vedas* and numerous important yoga texts, various references to *prana* and *pranayama* are made and their spiritual benefits are reflected upon. The sacred books of India are full of teachings on and references to the importance of *prana* and *pranayama*:

Mastery of pranayama removes the veil covering the light of knowledge and heralds the dawn of wisdom.
YOGA SUTRA

14
Unitive Paths for Living in the East and West

SANTOSHAN

If you were to speak about having an interest in yoga, a large majority of people would automatically think you were only talking about various postures, stretches and physical exercises associated with what is an immensely rich and vibrant tradition. It is odd that outside most yoga circles so little is known about other practices, especially as four principal yoga teachers who have had a huge impact on the West – Vivekananda, Yogananda, Aurobindo and Ramana Maharshi – are not particularly known for teachings on posture work.

Many routes and many choices
Looked at as a whole, and in its most inclusive form, yoga is about discovering what is suitable for our needs, nature and development, bringing peace and balance to our lives, and achieving positive and healthy development of the complete personality. This encompasses not only physical empowerment, but also mental, emotional and spiritual growth and maturity, which it should be noted, is not about a total self-reliance and an escape from life, but accepting and refining our human nature and the times when we need the support of friends.

Becoming more compassionate towards ourselves and others, maintaining awareness, performing right actions – in thought, word and deed – and attaining insight, wisdom and freedom from past conditioning can all be seen as important and linked facets of the universal message of yoga. It should also be pointed that yoga is not necessarily about religion or God, particularly from a monotheistic sense of God sitting in judgment, though it is often bound up with religious beliefs and practices. Patanjali's *Raja Yoga*, for instance, is actually classified as a philosophy, and like other yogas that link with or incorporate aspects of its teachings, it displays a deep psychological understanding of various levels of consciousness. A belief in God is not particularly prominent in the *Sutra*, but it could be argued that it was taken for granted and therefore did not need to be mentioned in detail. However, the various paths of yoga can be seen to focus on different types of practice that are undertaken in order to discover and reflect our true and authentic spiritual nature, which for some practitioners, can be done to achieve more of an existential transcendence without a particular belief in any Divine Principle.

Some possible early influences

Before we go any further, let us get back to the most known area of yoga, which is the unique physical posture work (*asanas*), which is primarily part of the hatha yoga tradition – the main manuals for which were written somewhere between the 6th and 15th centuries CE. The hatha yoga that we know today arose from the Tantric tradition. The Nath yogis (Tantric masters of yoga) are credited with developing it between the 8th and 11th centuries CE, though there are aspects of it which are much older. How far back some of the exercises go can only be speculated. Although scholars have found links between Tantra and some of the oldest Hindu rituals, it also displays elements that are unique to the tradition. Strong devotion to male and female deities, which initially appears to have grown more outside of Brahmanical/orthodox Hinduism, are predominantly featured. The early Vedic gods were predominantly male and had to be appeased.

It is possible that elements of hatha yoga emerged and were later blended with other exercises in the Hindu spiritual tradition, out of the practices of early wandering ascetics in India. Some early ascetics that are mentioned in the *Rig Veda* (Hinduism's oldest sacred teachings), which has sections that go back 3,500 years, are given the name 'munis'. Similar to the Nath yogis, they are credited with and described as having extraordinary powers.

Additionally, seals excavated from the Indus Valley sites, which flourished between 2500 and 1700 BCE, appear to show an early representation of the Hindu God Shiva, seated in a classic yogic position, with the soles of the feet touching each other. There has also been countless statues of the Mother Goddess found in the Indus Valley sites, which suggests that She must have been worship in almost every home.

Patanjali and hatha yoga

Some yogis claim that hatha yoga came out of Patanjali's *Yoga Sutra* with its influential eight-limbed path, but the only *asanas* mentioned in this work are sitting postures. Speculation hinges partly on the opening statement and the use of the word 'now' ('Now commences the exposition of yoga'), which appears to imply that it is building on other practices that are not written in the *Sutra* itself. As well as this, some of the exercises mentioned would usually be performed only after posture work.

An integrational approach

It is sometimes said that the three most popular yogas – jnana, karma and bhakti – aim at awakening to different aspects of the Divine: jnana to eternal pure being (*sat*), karma to the Divine Will (an aspect of pure consciousness: *chit*) and bhakti to pure bliss (*ananda*). However, the predominantly jnana yoga seers of the early *Upanishads* undermine this belief by realising Brahman, the Divine, as all three.

These days I feel the most complete and pragmatic approach to yoga is one of integration – transforming and harmonising the whole of what we are in order to awaken to and embody healthier states of being and understanding, which obviously includes our Supreme Nature, as well as our individual and social levels of being.

Swamiji herself, is known for encouraging a wide view of development that aims to work with all levels and achieve perfect equanimity between everyday life and spiritual living – to see all as sacred and every facet of ourselves as part of a spiritual whole. This can also be seen as the central message of Sri Aurobindo's integral approach. In many ways he was decades ahead of his time. Whether he was completely right about a current universal descent of the supermind bringing about a new era of spirituality remains to be seen, although the emergence of various inclusive paths to spirituality in recent years could be interpreted as a sign of its influence. For many yogis, however, this is the *kali-yuga* age: a time of decline. My personal belief is that the Divine is always creating and drawing us towards Its eternal goodness; even though we may not always be open to Its influence.

In writing about the process of transformation, Sri Aurobindo mentioned three essential points that actually stand in stark contrast to more systematic and world renouncing teachings. The following statement of Sri Aurobindo is quoted by Peter Heehs in his detailed biography of him (brackets are Peter Heehs's):

> *In the first place [the higher nature] does not act according to a fixed system and succession as in specialised methods of Yoga, but within a sort of free, scattered and yet gradually intensive and purposeful working determined by the temperament of the individual in whom it operates....*
>
> *Secondly, the process, being integral, accepts our nature such as it stands organised by our past evolution and without rejecting anything essential compels all to undergo a divine change....*
>
> *Thirdly, the divine Power in us uses all life as the means of this integral Yoga.*

One can see that there is a strong psychological aspect to Sri Aurobindo's yoga and this integrating of different disciplines is still happening today. Similar to Sri Aurobindo, many Western practitioners have combined aspects of yoga with modern psychotherapies. However, we should not think that this means ancient practices are being corrupted. It shows how vibrant and adaptable to today's needs yoga can be and is in many ways in-keeping with the tradition, as many of the exercises must surely have been arrived at through experimentation that tried different approaches which built on previous knowledge – just as there are people experimenting with the practices today which are building on previous knowledge.

The purpose of yoga

It is crucial to note that the word yoga translates as 'yoke', meaning to bind together and make whole. The word may also be translated as 'discipline' or 'union', which can be interpreted as the practice of unifying different parts of ourselves into a synthesized whole in order to overcome all sense of separation between the individual self and the Supreme Universal and Transcendent Self.

The body can be seen as the most sensible place for this transformation to begin and this is why hatha yoga has become an integral part of the tradition, though it is not always recognised as essential.

Yoga practitioners see the body as an important vehicle through which vital creative energy flows (*prana*). By implementing practices that the ancient tradition offers we become aware of this inherent power and energy and can then, through various exercises, find ways of using it to achieve healthier living. It is invariably seen as the starting place to awaken to and work with numerous levels of our being, including transforming levels of refined spiritual consciousness.

Pathways of yoga

The following is a brief description of some of the principal practices and branches of yoga. They should not be seen as isolated from one another; a combination of different elements will frequently be found within various schools. It is almost impossible to describe these paths and methods in just a few words. If you are seeking to further your knowledge and understanding of this tradition, there is a recommended reading section at the back of this book, which lists several primers on different types of yoga spirituality.

Bhakti yoga:	the path of devotion to God, seeing the Divine in all things and all people – unitive path of the heart.
Dhyana yoga:	the path of meditation – unitive path of focusing the mind and contemplative awareness.
Hatha yoga:	the path of physical postures and practices (part of Kundalini and Tantra yoga) – unitive path of the body.
Modern Integral yoga:	the synthesised path of self-discovery and expression formulated by Sri Aurobindo – unitive path of perfection, bhakti, jnana and karma yoga, which aims for a spiritual purification and transformation of the complete personality while living and acting in the world.

Jnana yoga: the path of intuitive knowledge and seeing beyond conditioned existence – unitive path of insight and wisdom.

Karma yoga: the path of work, good deeds and fulfiling one's obligations – unitive path of skilful and mindful action and use of the will.

Kundalini yoga: the path of awakening the active Shakti energy and rejoining it with the Absolute Consciousness – unitive path of the subtle body and psychic energy.

Mantra yoga: the path of recitation of sacred words and sounds – unitive path of sounds and vibrations.

Raja yoga: a psychological path that includes ethical precepts accredited to Patanjali (also called *Classical Yoga* and the *Yoga Sutra*) – unitive path of the mind and stages of progression.

Samkhya yoga: the path of analytical insight into the nature of the world and the transcendent Self, which was systemised by Ishvara Krishna – unitive path of philosophy.

Tantra yoga: the path of guru and student initiation into yoga (the chakras and kundalini energy are a part of this tradition) – unitive path of the transformation of base energies.

Additionally, Kriya yoga (the yoga of ritual action) can refer to either Raga yoga or practices associated with Kundalini yoga.

Yoga in the *Gita*

The *Bhagavad Gita* (the Song of the Blessed One) starts with a dialogue between the warrior prince Arjuna and the revered Divine figure Krishna that takes place on the eve of a great battle. It is, perhaps, the most loved of all Hindu scriptures, written in poetic verse and placed as part of the *Mahabharata*: a key text in the Hindu tradition. The battle has been interpreted as symbolic by various yoga teachers and is seen as being linked with different aspects of spiritual unfoldment.

The *Gita* urges everyone to take up yoga and practise it as an essential part of their lives and that various paths be combined into one complete system. Within this are included four principal paths of yoga that are fundamentally bound-up with ideas about the Divine:

(1) The path of surrender of one's self and all actions to the Divine (God-centred karma yoga).
(2) The path of knowledge of the true Self and its oneness in the Divine (God-centred jnana yoga).
(3) The path of devotion and love of God (bhakti yoga).
(4) The path of meditation and awareness of the Divine (God-centred dhyana yoga).

Additionally, there are aspects of Raga and Samkhya yoga that can be found in parts of the *Gita's* overall synthesis, such as the observance of various virtues, the understanding of different forces that work within us, and the elements and psychological levels of ourselves. But the *Gita* does not take the same route as Raga and Samkhya yoga. The *Gita's* central message of devotion and involvement in the world it not so predominant in Raga yoga, and Samkhya is more coldly analytical in its approach and believes in many separate Spirit-Selves (*purushas*), without any clear concept of God – though the *Gita* itself, also draws upon rational observations and encourages reflective thinking about various areas of development.

The *Gita* and devotional yoga

The *Gita's* treatise on karma yoga is considered sublime, but above all it is its verses on devotion which have made it so popular. It is seen as the vital ingredient to attaining salvation. Through devotion to God we come to know the Divine more intimately:

By love he knows me in truth, who I am and what I am.
And when he knows me in truth he enters into my Being.

In its purest form, devotion takes on a universal approach to spiritual development, by loving and worshipping all life, things and people as part of the Divine; for if all is grounded in the Oneness of God, then all can equally be worshiped as God. Yet followers of devotional yoga will generally and more obviously revere the Divine in a personal form, through which they may find a unity with an impersonal and more abstract truth. It depends on the approach and one's belief and experience. For non-dual Vedantists, the Ultimate is traditionally without form and non-personal, whereas for bhakti followers there is a personal Creator who eternally loves us. Yet, there are rainbows within rainbows of belief within all traditions and even India's greatest non-dual Vedantist philosopher Shankara was a devout follower of the Hindu God Shiva all his life.

The *Gita* and intuitive wisdom

Teachings about jnana yoga in the *Gita* aim to encourage us to see intuitively through the dualities of nature and the universe in order to reach a point of seeing and understanding all as a manifestation of the Divine – as God permeates the seen and unseen. Behind the appearance of the many there is One Divine Creative Cause of all.

In the *Gita*, Krishna describes his Divine nature as follows, in which both intuitive spiritual knowledge and the experience and workings of nature are seen as part of His omnipresent Power:

> *I am the taste of living waters and the light of the sun and the moon ...*
> *... Of all knowledge I am the knowledge of the Soul. Of the many paths of reason I am the one that leads to truth.*

Jnana yoga is a path for those with discriminating insight who can wisely perceive the Ultimate Reality within and beyond the world. Within the *Gita* there are many references to the path of spiritual knowledge and discrimination, but it is generally integrated as a part of the *Gita's* own unique synthesis.

The *Gita* and the path of action

More than any other form of practice, karma yoga is perhaps the most practical of all, as it deals with the problems of living, the creative uses of the will and with our actions having consequences.

The principal teachings on karma yoga in the *Gita* are about non-attachment for the purpose of overcoming restrictive actions and doing everything as an offering to God – so linking ethical conduct strongly with devotional yoga.

The *Gita* reminds us that through non-attachment we find reward by losing our sense of separation from the Divine and discover freedom within that unity: "for performing actions without attachment man and woman attains the highest." This is seen as a way of acting selflessly and skilfully in the world and, as a practice whereby one overcomes strong associations with conditioned existence and consequently starts to live a purer life:

> *Offer all thy works to God, throw off selfish bonds, and do thy work.*
> *No sin can stain thee, even as waters do not stain the leaf of the lotus.*

The *Gita* and the path of meditation

The *Gita* combines both discipline and meditation together, for without discipline meditation would be impossible, as we would never be able to keep the body and mind still.

Krishna encourages Arjuna to see life non-dualistically, by advising him to take the same mental stand towards good and evil – a form of watching the mind without judgment that connects with the witness consciousness and the discerning wisdom of jnana yoga. Other meditation practices are mentioned, such as breathing exercises, sensual withdrawal, concentration, chanting, focusing the mind on a single object and gazing at the tip of the nose. Paramahansa Yogananda claimed the latter to be wrongly understood by translators and states in his *Autobiography of a Yogi* that it refers to the point between the eyebrows, i.e. the bridge of the nose.

The synthesis of the *Gita*

We have seen how various practices and beliefs are discussed in the *Gita* and their merits reflected upon. But it is the *Gita's* own integral devotional approach, intrinsically bound-up with karma yoga and ethical, non-violent and compassionate conduct, along with aspects of jnana yoga and meditation that ultimately wins the day:

> *Doing My work, intent on Me, devoted to Me, free from attachment,*
> *free from enmity to all beings, who is so, comes to Me ...*

Today, we might argue the merits of other paths. But we should remember that no practice advocated in the *Gita* is seen in isolation. Nonetheless, some might agree that love more than any other attribute, when expanded to embrace all life and people (as the *Gita* advocates), is the highest quality humankind possesses. For the philosopher Roy Bhaskar, as well as other numerous teachers of wisdom, philosophy and spirituality, love is the most uniting, healing, expanding and energising force in the universe.

Where do we go from here?

Within this book Swamiji and I have explored and shared various thoughts about the richness of the yogic tradition, as well as other ancient and contemporary perspectives on spirituality. All could be considered as a finger pointing to the moon, and as the Zen saying goes, it is obviously foolish to mistake the finger for the moon. Yet to dismiss any wisdom is to overlook the Creativity of the Divine revealing Itself in different ways within our world and cosmos. Just as we find a sense of the sacred in the awe we experience when seeing beauty in a setting sun, there is as much sacred and deep beauty in spiritual insights and teachings that remind us profoundly of our true nature.

All paths have merit if followed with compassion and wisdom. Yoga has discovered many great truths to live by. But there are areas it has not fully explored, and has at times dismissed or overlooked, and that is why references have been made in this book to other traditions – both ancient and modern – which I hope has helped to add another dimension it. The search needs to go on continuously, as every age has different needs and values, which are forever changing. We do not even look at the world in the same way that our grandparents did when they were our age. Scientifically, culturally, sociologically, politically, psychologically and morally we have changed and have a different understanding about life and spirituality. The paths we tread must be relevant to the world we live in now. Yoga, in its most universal form, includes all facets of ourselves as a means for transformation and spiritual empowerment. If this book has encouraged a more inclusiveness, then some of the reasons for putting it together have been justified. For today's world and its inhabitants require us all to live our beliefs to their most all-embracing. This must be the yoga that we practise today. If it is not, then we should ask why this is so.

PART FOUR
Further Exercises

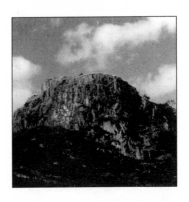

*Let us all continue to grow in love, wisdom and the Spirit,
and to share our growth with each other.*
SWAMI DHARMANANDA

*We must endeavour to unite and serve humanity
in and through love, peace, harmony and friendship.*
SANTOSHAN

Be still and know. Remain in a state of spiritual wakefulness,
with your mind and senses open, to hear what God wills in every moment.
ABBOT VASILIOS

In stillness we not only find our individual self,
but we find our Universal Self,
for the extent of every man is vast as the Universe.
The entire Universe is within each and everyone.
It is only when the individuality merges away in Universality that
we become boundless and timeless and experience that all is One.
GURURAJ ANANDA

It is said that when you take only one step towards Him,
He advances ten steps towards you.
But the complete truth is that God is always with you.
MUHAMMAD

If even only for a moment you can throw yourself into That in which
there are no separate beings, then you will hear what God says.
Just stop all your thinking and willing,
and you will hear the unspeakable words of God.
JACOB BOEHME

Wherever there is sincerity and goodwill, the Divine's help also is there.
THE MOTHER
(MIRA ALFASSA)

15

Nadi Shodhana Practices

SWAMI DARMANANDA

The practice of *nadi shodhana* is for purification of the *pranic* passages (*nadis*), thus enabling the *prana* (vital force) to flow freely. It is considered to be an excellent preparation for meditation techniques.

> *Nadi* = Psychic passage. The *nadis* are channels, which are said to conduct vital energy throughout the body.
> *Shodhana* = Purification, cleansing.

Sit in a position you can hold comfortably, with the spine erect. Practise breath awareness until the breath is steady, then start *nadi shodhana* Stage 1.

Stage 1: first practice

Hold the right hand in front of the face and place the index finger and middle fingers on the forehead between the eyebrows. Rest the thumb on the right nostril and the ring finger on the left nostril. The little finger is left free. This is known as the *nasagra mudra*.

1. Exhale through both nostrils.

2. Gently close the right nostril with the thumb.

3. Inhale and exhale through the left nostril five times.

4. Release the pressure of the thumb and gently close the left nostril with the ring finger.

5. Inhale and exhale through the right nostril five times.

6. Release the *nasagra mudra* and breathe through both nostrils five times.

This constitutes one round. Establish this practice over a period of weeks so that you can do five rounds comfortably before proceeding to the next practice.

Stage 1: second practice
Inhale and exhale through both nostrils to a count of five seconds. Establish this rhythm and then apply the *nasagra mudra*.

1. Close the right nostril and inhale through the left nostril for a count of five seconds. Exhale though the left nostril for a count of five seconds.

2. Release the right nostril and close the left nostril. Inhale through the right nostril for a count of five seconds. Exhale through the right nostril for a count of five seconds.

3. Complete the round by inhaling and exhaling through both nostrils for a count of five seconds.

You could start with one round and gradually increase until you can perform five rounds comfortably and with complete awareness of the process of 'observing the breath'.

Stage 1: third practice
Establish the previous practice over a period of weeks before proceeding with the following:

1. Inhale and exhale through both nostrils.

2. Apply the *nasagra mudra*, closing the nostrils as in the previous practice.

3. Inhale to a count of five seconds through the left nostril.

4. Exhale to a count of five seconds through the right nostril.

5. Inhale to a count of five seconds through the right nostril.

6. Exhale to a count of five seconds through the left nostril.

This is one round. Continue practising alternate nostril breathing for as long as it is comfortable. It is best to start with five rounds and then gradually build up to ten if comfortable.

Although these are the basic practices, if they are done on a regular basis (even for only ten minutes a day) they can be powerful instruments for bringing about a purification and harmony between the body, emotions, mind and Spirit.

Precautions and practical advice
• You must stop any practice if discomfort is felt.
• There must be no strain either physical or mental.
• Make preliminary preparations, such as making sure your seat is comfortable, the is body relaxed and the back is upright.
• The posture should be held without strain.
• Light non-restrictive clothing should be worn, with no restrictions round the waist or abdomen.
• It is a good idea to wrap a shawl or blanket around oneself in case the body temperature drops.
• The room should be well ventilated, but warm and free from draughts.
• You will need quiet, and conditions which will not distract or disturb your concentration.
• Early morning or the evening are very suitable times. But everyone must choose a time that is suitable for their lifestyle.
• Try and practise at the same time each day if possible.
• Do not practise immediately after a meal and do not eat until at least half an hour after practice. With extensive practise a light diet is preferable. If combined with other practices, breathing techniques

should come after physical exercise and before meditation.

• Breathing should be through the nose and not through the mouth unless otherwise stated.

• High blood pressure and heart disease should be taken into account. If in any doubt consult a medical practitioner. For advanced practices consult an experienced teacher.

• It is advocated that all breathing exercises should be slowly and systematically developed.

• Violent respiration is to be avoided. The lungs should be treated with respect. Full use of the lungs, intercostal muscles and diaphragm should be encouraged by controlling respiration, without strain

• Work towards a harmonisation of the whole self: the body, the mind, the emotions and the Spirit.

Stage 2: first practice

Sit in a position you can hold comfortably, with the spine erect. Practise breath awareness until the rhythm of the breath is steady. Establish alternate nostril breathing, as in Stage 1, before proceeding:

1. Inhale and exhale through both nostrils.

2. Apply the *nasagra mudra* (using the finger and thumb of the right hand to control the breath flow).

3. Inhale to a count of five seconds through the left nostril.

4. Exhale to a count of five seconds through the right nostril.

5. Inhale to a count of five seconds through the right nostril.

6. Exhale to a count of five seconds through the left nostril.

This is one round. Practise five to ten rounds and establish over a period of weeks before moving on.

Stage 2: second practice

Increase the exhalation by one second (outlined below).

1. Inhale for five seconds.

2. Exhale for six seconds.
If this is comfortable, then gradually increase the exhalation until it is twice as long as the inhalation, i.e.

1. Inhale for five seconds.

2. Exhale for ten seconds.

Practise five to ten rounds and establish over a period of weeks before moving onto Stage 3. If you wish to practise the following breathing techniques, it will be advisable to find an experienced teacher for proper guidance, particularly for longer retention of the breath.

Stage 3: first practice

Sit down and give yourself time to establish a comfortable posture, with the spine erect. Practise breath awareness until the rhythm of the breath is steady. Establish alternate nostril breathing as described in Stage 1 and Stage 2. Proceed as follows:

1. Inhale through the left nostril for a count of four seconds.

2. Retain the in-breath for four seconds.

3. Exhale through the right nostril for a count of eight seconds.

4. Inhale through the right nostril for a count of four seconds.

5. Retain the in-breath for four seconds.

6. Exhale through the left nostril for a count of eight seconds.

This constitutes one round. Make sure the exhalation is steady, not rushed or strained. If you find that a steady exhalation is difficult after retention of the breath, shorten the time of exhalation to four seconds, then gradually increase until the out-breath is twice as long as the in-breath. Begin with five rounds and gradually increase to ten if comfortable. Practise over a period of weeks before moving onto the next exercise

Stage 3: second practice

Gradually increase breath retention until you can retain the breath for four times as long as you take to inhale, i.e.

1. Inhalation = four seconds.   (1)

2. Retention = sixteen seconds.   (4)

3. Exhalation = eight seconds.   (2)

Those who become proficient in this practice may lengthen the inhalation, retention and exhalation. But do not attempt to do so if you find it difficult.

Note

The practices in this book are simple, but as stated before they have powerful effects. It is suggested that they be practised consistently and their effects and benefits are understood before they are passed on.

16
Body, Feelings, Mind

SANTOSHAN

BODY	FEELINGS
MIND	

For the following exercise you will need a selection of coloured crayons and a large sheet of white paper, approximately 420 x 300 mm (18 x 15 inches) or bigger. This exercise is more effective when it is done quickly – but not rushed – as it stops the rational mind from interfering with any intuitive insights that emerge:

1. Divide the paper into four sections and write the word 'body' in one section, then 'feelings' in another, and 'mind' in a third section. You should end up with something that looks like the diagram above.

2. Sit quietly with your eyes closed. Relax the body and remain still and quiet for a few minutes.

3. Become aware of your physical body. Feel the weight of your body upon the chair or cushion you are sitting on. Become aware of your inhaling and exhaling breath and of the rhythm of your breath. Even though you are now relaxed, notice if there are any physical sensations or if there is any tension in your body.

4. Notice whether there is a specific area that draws your attention to it and observe the sensation. Notice if the sensation is cold, hot, warm, comforting, irritating, painful or constricting, or whether it is another type of sensation. Stay with the sensation for a moment and see what emerges from it. Ask yourself what your body is trying to tell you. What is behind the sensation?

5. When you are ready, open your eyes and choose whatever coloured crayons attract your attention and draw the sensation (or sensations) that emerged. Draw in whatever style you find the easiest and free-flowing, using either abstract shapes and/or pictures. You may also wish to include some words with your drawing.

6. Put your drawing aside for a moment and sit quietly again. This time, become aware of any feelings or emotions. Notice whatever feelings or emotions emerge. Ask yourself what type of feelings and/ or emotions they are. Are they pleasant or unpleasant, uplifting or depleting, positive or negative? Ask yourself what these feelings or emotions are about?

7. When you are ready, draw whatever feelings or emotions you became aware of in the appropriate section.

8. Put your drawing aside for a moment and sit quietly again. Now take your attention to your mind and its thoughts. Become aware of any thoughts, impressions or mental images that you have.

9. When you are ready, draw any thoughts, impressions and images that you became aware of in the appropriate section of the paper.

10. Now look at your three drawings and see what they tell you about yourself. Ask yourself what area is the most predominant. Are you more predominantly strong in the thinking, feeling or physical area?

Many people are surprise at what emerges at this stage.

Ask yourself if there is any area that is calling for more attention than others, and ask what this part of you needs. Ask yourself what you need to do to take care of this part of yourself. See what emerges and write your feelings, thoughts, impressions and intuitions in the remaining section of the paper.

Further exercise: peeling away the body, feelings and mind

1. Sit quietly and become aware of different parts of your being. Become aware of your physical body, your feelings and of any thoughts that surface. Stay with them for a short while and then allow them to fall away – rather like peeling away layers of an onion.

2. Slowly disidentify from each layer of your physical, emotional and mental self and realise they are only parts of a greater whole. Realise that behind each layer there is a larger experience of spaciousness that has the ability to heal all inhibiting wounds and lead you to larger possibilities of being.

Gently become aware of your breath and its natural rhythm, and allow it to help you to let go of your physical, emotional and mental self and lead you to a more open state of being that knows no limitations. Just go with the experience and stay with it for as long as it feels natural and comfortable. Be present in the experience without imposing any preconceptions about how it will happen or where it will take you. Just be open, receptive and fully present to the experience.

3. When you feel ready to come back, consciously feel an embodiment of the expanded state that you have awakened to. Notice how it has lightened your physical being, clarified your thoughts, loosened up any tension or inhibiting emotions. Notice how your feelings are now more positive, how your mind is more creative and awake, and how your physical body feels more healed, balanced and refreshed.

Realise that this experience is not temporary and that you have brought something to the surface of your being that has always been there, which you have now made a more active influence in your life and spiritual development.

4. Finish with an affirmation, such as the following one, that acknowledges the changes you have brought about:

I am open and receptive to the creative influence of the infinite Self.
I live harmoniously with all life that surrounds me
and with all life within me.

APPENDIX I
Hindu Wisdom

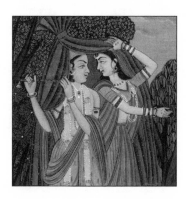

*Yoga practices are about the inward journey towards
truth, knowledge, understanding and wisdom,
and the joining of our individual being
with the Divine Light of God.*
SWAMI DHARMANANDA

*The wisdom of the past is always with us; it is eternal.
Look within and you will discover it for yourself.*
SANTOSHAN

I have tasted the sweet drink of life, knowing that it inspires good thoughts
and joyous expansiveness to the extreme ... When you penetrate inside, you
will know no limitations ...
RIG VEDA

Words cannot describe the joy of the soul whose impurities are cleansed
in deep contemplation – who is one with his atman, his own Spirit.
MAITRI UPANISHAD

Do thy work in the peace of yoga and, free from selfish desires,
be not moved in success or in failure.
Yoga is evenness of mind – a peace that is ever the same.
BHAGAVAD GITA

Like the sun the Self is one.
But like the sun reflected on moving water
the Self appears to be broken into many forms.
But I learned from the sun
not to mistake the image for the reality.
UDDHAVA GITA

No matter what he is doing – walking, standing, sitting or lying down – the
illumined seer whose delight is the atman lives in joy and freedom.
CREST-JEWEL OF WISDOM

Sitting
Down Near

SWAMI DARMANANDA and SANTOSHAN

Lead me from the unreal to the Real
Lead me from darkness to the Light.
Lead me from death to immortality.
BRHADARANYAKA UPANISHAD

The word 'Upanishad' is seen to roughly translate as 'sitting down near', implying the practice of being close to one's spiritual teacher in order to hear his or her words of wisdom. It can also be broken down as follows:

UPA   a competent teacher
NI   loosens/destroys
SHAD   attachment

The rise of mystical insight

A growing debate has arisen about the beginnings of the Hindu spiritual tradition. One particular view that has caused controversy is that around the middle of the 2nd millennium BCE nomadic tribes calling themselves 'Aryans' (the noble ones), began to spread out from somewhere beyond the North-West regions of Asia. Some of these tribes it is said made their way into the Indian sub-continent where the Indus Valley Civilisation existed, which dates back to around 2500 BCE and disintegrated around 1700 BCE.

Many hotly debate the belief about the Aryans coming from outside of India. Perhaps the only sensible answer is to say that no one knows for sure, as there currently appears to be no satisfactory evidence which everyone agrees upon. However, everyone at least seems to be in agreement about the Indus Valley Civilisation.

Within the Indus Valley there was a thriving community, advanced in technology and trade, with a remarkable method of irrigation, water preservation, drainage and even a flushing sewage system, who lived peacefully with one another and in harmony with nature. What is known about the Aryan people, who followed the practices of the *Vedas* (Hinduism's oldest sacred teachings), is that they had strong religious beliefs in many gods, their own particular forms of worship and their own priests (brahmins) who conducted various rituals.

It is thought, on the one hand, that there was an amalgamation of these two people's beliefs – Aryan and Indus – which happened over a period of time. On the other hand, it is believed that the Indus people were in fact the Aryans. But as very little is known about the Indus Valley people and the Aryans themselves, we can, perhaps, only speculate about these views and hope that evidence will soon emerge to settle matters.

Seals have been discovered in the ancient sites of the Indus Valley depicting a male figure in a yogic sitting position, which some have considered to be an early depiction of the Hindu God Shiva. They have also uncovered a particular large water tank structure, which appears to have been used for ritual purposes, as is sometimes used in the Hindu tradition today.

From the early *Vedas* to the *Upanishads*

Eventually the *Vedas* (also called *Samhitas*), four collections of ancient and sacred knowledge and practices, appeared: the *Rig*, *Yajur*, *Sama* and *Atharva*. What is known is that hymns and rituals of the *Vedas* were adopted by the people populating various regions that now make up the Indian sub-continent.

The *Rig Veda* is the oldest – although recent scholarship has argued that there are portions of the *Atharva Veda* which are as old as some sections of the *Rig Veda*. But generally, the other *Vedas* are seen to follow in the order mentioned above from the *Rig Veda*. They contain prayers, hymns, chants and rituals (symbolic sacrifice), which form part of the Hindu tradition. They also contain some commentaries, made by the brahmin priests, explaining the ancient rites. The *Atharva Veda* contains more magical incantations than instruction for orthodox rituals and practices, which appear to be moving towards the religion of the ordinary people.

The *Vedas,* along with other early teachings, were remembered by using various means of meter, sound and repetition and handed down aurally until a system of writing was developed. The Indus Valley people did have a form of writing, which was unfortunately lost when the civilisation went into decline. It remains the only undeciphered ancient language left in the world.

The word 'Veda' comes from the root word *vid,* meaning 'to know'. The teachings of the *Vedas* are seen as revealed sacred knowledge (*sruti*), of which the *Upanishads* are also part of. Modern scholarship dates the earliest *Upanishads* – *Brhadaranyaka* and *Chandogya* – to around 800 BCE. The *Upanishads* are considered to be the end of the *Vedas.* The *Brahmanas* (which describe various rituals) and the *Aranyakas* (supplementary teachings for forest hermits) fall in-between the four *Vedas* and the *Upanishads.*

Whereas the first part of the Vedic teachings focus on exterior rituals relevant to the Vedic religion, the last part – the *Upanishads* – is concerned with meditative practices and mystical wisdom which is universally applicable. Rituals are usually only appropriate to a particular culture, period of history or belief, but spiritual wisdom can be as appropriate today as it ever was.

The background to the teachers of the *Upanishads* is not absolutely clear. It has been suggested that they were men and women who retired to the forests for the purpose of attaining mystical insights. The *Aranyakas* may have opened up the way and made the ground more fertile for the universal message of the *Upanishads* to be accepted.

Pantheistic leanings of the *Upanishads* can be seen to link with the *Artharva Veda* and the *Brahmanas.* The symbolism of the early Vedic literature is also invariably drawn upon. But on the whole, the *Upanishads* take a different stand. The famous 'That thou art' (*tat tvam asi*) from the *Chandogya Upanishad,* points to a Reality that is both 'One and Many', beyond all forms and appearances: One into which the mystic merges.

Although some ideas can be found in the *Brahmanas,* they do not share the experiential and mystical ideas of the *Upanishads* and do not come to the conclusion that *atman* is Brahman. Academic research believes the *Upanishads* show an outside influence coming in. The fact that some of the teachers of the *Upanishads* are not from the usual priest caste and are women shows that something different is happening. Additionally there are key teachings which were not there before.

Just how many of the *Classical Upanishads* were composed and handed down is not known. It is said to be thousands. But a hundred and eight is often an accepted number – no doubt because of it being a sacred number (there are a hundred and eight prayer beads on Hindu and Buddhist *malas*). The great Vedantin philosopher Shankara (788-820CE) revived interest in the teachings by writing commentaries on around ten of the *Upanishads*. It is suggested that he commented on others, but they have been lost.

More recently, scholars have commentated on and translated other *Upanishads*, and today we have access to these translations, so we can read the words of wisdom spoken by the wise men and women who taught over two thousand years ago, and can be inspired by their sacred knowledge. There have been other *Upanishads* written over the years, but they are not seen as part of the early classical teachings.

The list below shows eleven early *Upanishads* which are generally considered to be the most important. Each one is placed with one of the four *Vedas*, as shown in brackets. They are still used today and are among the most popular and influential. The *Svetasvatara* is one of the *Upanishads* that scholars believe Shankara wrote a commentary for, but was lost – only part of the work was found. The *Svetasvatara Upanishad* is an important early devotional work which was written around the time of the *Bhagavad Gita* and most likely predates it.

ELEVEN PRINCIPAL UPANISHADS

Brhadaranyaka (White Yajur Veda)	Taittiriya (Black Yajur Veda)
Mandukya (Atharva Veda)	Prashna (Atharva Veda)
Kena (Sama Veda)	Chandogya (Sama Veda)
Katha (Black Yajur Veda)	Isha (White Yajur Veda)
Mundaka (Atharva Veda)	Svetasvatara (Black Yajur)
Aitareya (Rig Veda)	

Breaking new ground

There is no single authorship, cohesive theme or one system of philosophy and practice that runs through the whole of the *Classical Upanishads*. Early ones, such as the *Brhadaranyaka* and *Chandogya*, which are considered the most historically important, teach monistic ideas about Brahman (the Divine).

There has been a tendency to see that what is taught today is exactly the same as the *Upanishads* and the four *Vedas*. But this misses out on acknowledging the richness of different beliefs, practices and insights that have emerged. Within the early *Upanishads* there is a shift from ideas about various devas and Vedic rituals and sacrifices, to meditation, mystical experience and more sophisticated beliefs about the Self and the One behind the multiple forms of Creation – both seen and unseen:

> *In the highest golden sheath is Brahman without stain,*
> *without parts;*
> *Pure is it, the light of lights.*
> *That is what the knowers of Self know.*
> MUNDAKA UPANISHAD

The absolute monism of later Advaita Vedanta philosophy is not arrived at in the early teachings. It is the relatively late *Mundaka Upanishad* that begins to display it. But one passage where the Imperishable/Ultimate and Creation are compared to a spider weaving its web and plants sprouting from the earth, suggests that the world and Brahman are not completely identical.

Nonetheless, major concepts are introduced and developed which display a new understanding of the human condition and of salvation, such as karma, the cycle of lives (*samsara*), personal liberation (*moksha*), desires inhibiting our spiritual growth and humankind living in blindness of its true nature. Yoga writer Georg Feuerstein mentions in his book *Wholeness or Transcendence?* that a few hymns of the *Rig Veda* seem to indicate some previous knowledge of reincarnation, but the full fleshing out of its teachings is not done until the later *Upanishads*.

From the time of the early *Upanishads* onwards most of these ideas remain central not only to Hindu and yogic teachings, but many other spiritual traditions that emerged in India. Where these insights came from can only be speculated. Some have suggested they could have come from an influential tribal religion, which the teachers of the *Upanishads* were in contact with.

Freedom from conditioned existence

A key point is that the *atman* (man's and woman's inner essence) is seen as immortal and as Brahman, the ground of everything and everyone. Those who have insight into this Reality know their true Self:

> *He or She, Knower of the Self*
> *Reaches 'That' highest plane of Brahman*
> *In which all is contained*
> *And shines brightly.*
> MUNDAKA UPANISHAD

This is an awakening to a transcendent and omnipresent Reality which is realised in higher states of meditation and is different from early Vedic ideas about the soul, as they were more bound-up with notions of ancestor worship. Liberation from conditioned existence and the world of change and unsatisfactoriness (the world of *samsara*) is the prime focus of the Upanishadic teachers. This is not seen as a way of blissing-out and escaping from the world, but more of a positive help to living life more peacefully.

Mystical Knowledge

It can be argued that the road to the experiential and meditative aspect of the *Upanishads* was already open through the taking of *soma* (an hallucinogenic substance) in the early Vedic period. But by the time of the *Upanishads* the practice had died out and the ingredients were forgotten. Nonetheless, it shows that we are dealing with a culture that was receptive to ideas and practices connected with altered-states of consciousness.

In the *Upanishads*, normal states of mind have to be transcended in order to awaken to the Ultimate Reality/Brahman, which is said to be in a fourth state of existence (normal consciousness, dreams and dreamless sleep being the other three). Brahman pervades all things and is the true Self which has always existed, unbound and unaffected by time, action, decay, death or physical conditions.

The expression *neti, neti*, which is more accurately translated as 'not, not', illustrates that both *atman* and Brahman are something so 'totally other' than anything normally perceived in life. It is, therefore, easier to describe what they are not than what they are. But this does not imply a state of nothingness. The closest expression offered to describe Brahman is, 'pure being, pure consciousness, pure bliss' (*sat-chit-ananda*).

Karma in the *Upanishads*

There are two aspects to karma: one positive (*punya*) and one negative (*papa*). The *Upanishads* introduce the idea of a subtle body which stores up karma and determines and influences one's present or future life. Good deeds are advocated, as this determines a better rebirth. But to achieve complete freedom from the cycle of rebirth, non-attachment to all worldly actions is recommended. This does not imply uninvolvement in the world. We must remember that some of the teachers of the *Upanishads* are married and in contact with others – they are not reclusive ascetics. Those who pursue earthly desire are seen to be bound by their actions, whereas those who desire only Brahman find both freedom in this life and the next.

In the early *Upanishads* salvation is attained through overcoming a lack of awareness of one's true nature and seeing the world as neither good nor bad. The Upanishadic road to freedom is a path of intuitively seeing beyond dualities – realising the whole universe and beyond as Brahman and knowing that That Reality is also part of oneself:

Oh Supreme Spirit –
Nourisher,
Controller of all,
Illuminating Light,
Fountain of Life
For all beings – Withhold thy binding light,

Gather in thy rays,
So we may see,
Through thy Grace
The blessed formulation,
The Divine,
That which dwells within us,
Is 'That Being' 'That' am I.
ISHA UPANISHAD*

*Main quotations of the *Upanishads* are from Alan Jacobs's excellent translation, *The Principal Upanishads: A Poetic Translation* (O Books, 2003).

Popular Gods and Goddesses and Elements of Hinduism Chart

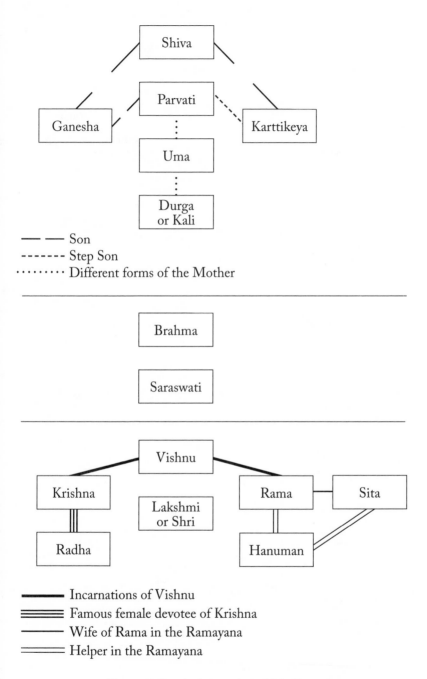

FIGURE 10: *Popular Puranic Gods and Goddesses*

ELEMENTS OF HINDUISM

Indus Valley

Between 2500 & 1700 BCE the first civilisation in Indian emerged with the cities of Harappa and Mohenjo-daro, separated by 400 miles. A third site has recently been discovered on an island.

The sites have a system of water preservation and a central tank structure that could have been used for ritual bathing: a feature in Hinduism to this day.

Speculations have been made about the Indus Valley people being Dravidian speaking tribes.

The Indus Valley sites show possible signs of male fertility rites, animal and nature worship, including trees, horned-oxen and snakes.
  Numerous terra-cotta statues of the Mother Goddess have also been unearthed, which suggests that She may have been worshipped in almost every home.

Unearthed objects from the sites resemble the shape of a lingam. There has also been the discovery of seals showing a figure seated in a yoga posture and has led some to speculated it as being an early depiction of the Hindu God Shiva.
  Most of the seals discovered include a script that has not yet been deciphered.

Note: Cross-fertilisation has occurred between the different categories.
  The word 'Hinduism' is an umbrella term for various beliefs and practices and comes from a word which was originally used to describe the Indian people.

Beginnings of Yoga?

Some of the seals found in the Indus Valley suggest some form of early yoga practice, but cannot be proven for sure.

Before the middle of the 1st millennium BCE there was a growing number of wandering ascetics. The *Rig Veda* X.136 describes long-haired ascetics called 'munis', who had extraordinary powers and went around naked or in soiled yellow garments. Similar to tribal shamans, they could fly through the air, perceive all forms and know the thoughts of others.

Tapas (internal heat) develops into notions about exposing oneself to pain. But asceticism had no place in the early Vedic framework and world renunciation is only placed as the last stage of life after the early *Upanishads*.

Breathing exercises *may* have evolved from the repetition of mantras.

Yoga meditation is mentioned in the *Upanishads*. The *Chandogya, Katha, Prasna* and *Maitri Upanishads* mention the *'nadis'* (psychic channels). The *Maitri Upanishad* has a six-limbed system of yoga and mentions *'susumna'* (a central psychic channel).

The *Yoga Sutra* has an eight-limbed system of breathing exercises, etc., but only mentions sitting postures. Speculation has arisen about it being used for teachings *after* yogic postures, as the practices mentioned are usually done today.

Between the 6th-15th century CE the main manuals of Hatha Yoga are compiled.

Vedic Period

People known as Aryans come to the fore around the 2nd millennium BCE. They speak Sanskrit, which goes out of popular use around 5th century BCE. They have an oral tradition with religious poems and hymns which are eventually cut down into mantras.

The four *Vedas* focus on outward ritual–a personal relationship with many devas/nature gods, but are not particularly devotional. There is no 'One God' with a capital 'G'. Rituals performed for victory in battle, etc.
  Brahman is mentioned, but is not the same as the *Upanishads'* view. It is more about the power embodied in the *Vedas*, of which a priest can tap into.
  The *Rig, Sama* and *Yajur Vedas* are for different priestly functions. The *Atharva Veda* is moving to the level of ordinary people (1st part as old as other *Vedas*) and are rituals you can do at home yourself. The *Rig Veda* (X:90) mentions four divisions of society.

The *Brahmanas* are later responses to the *Vedas*. They show a lot of myths starting to come in and a predominance of sacrifices. They describe rituals and how to perform them, i.e. say right hymns, make offerings to uphold cosmic order (*rita*)–a kind of early idea of karma.

Chapter X of the *Rig Veda* (which is a later section) and the *Brahmanas* outwardly speculate about a One behind the many.

The *Aranyakas* are ritual treatises for forest dwellers to reflect on and may have opened up some of the way for the *Upanishads*.

THE BRAHMANICAL TRADITION

PERIOD 3-4
The Upanishads

Early *Upanishads* (800 BCE), *Brihadaranyaka* and *Chandogya*, develop ideas about liberation, karma (desire in the early *Upanishads*) and *samsara* (cycle of lives and the human condition).

They show an outside influence coming in and introduce mystical experience, meditation and monistic ideas. Liberation is about self-effort and knowledge of the true Self. Some teachers are *kshatriyas* and are married, and some are women.

New *Upanishads* are written and the principal ones are collected together and reflected upon as a whole.

Later *Upanishads*, such as the *Svetasvatara*, personalise God and come up with a cohesive synthesis of yoga practices and an early form of *bhakti* (devotion). *Maitri Upanishad* mentions *ashramas* (stages of life) and fulfiling one's *svadharma* (personal duty).

PERIOD 4+
6 Classic Philosophies

Vaisesika and Nyaya are different to the other four, and historically of little importance.

Vaisesika: Oldest text and ideas pre-date other systems, but developed later in the 10th century CE. Starts as a primitive form of science, breaking things down into specific components. A kind of ancient cosmology and physics. Originally had no religious connections.

Nyaya: Starts in the area of logic–a debating technique.

Mimasa: Looks at a system of Vedic ritual and the four *Vedas* and how they are then split up. It tries to find an Original Source and questions the nature of things. Comes up with the idea of an eternal Veda which reveals itself. Not a 'Truth', but something a Hindu has to do: duty, etc. The *Dharma Shastras* were used as a link, but Mimasa holds no concept of God.

PERIOD 4+
Orthodox Developments

The *Law Books* (*Dharma Sutras* and *Dharma Shastras*), written by Brahmin priests, are arguably impossible to enforce on everyone. Key ideas are:

(a) General virtues for all: self-control, kindness, tell truth, etc.

(b) Notion of four stages of life (*ashramas*): 1. *Bramachary* (celibate student); 2. *Grhastha* (householder); 3. *Vanaprastra* (forest dweller); and 4. *Sannyasin* (renouncer of the world).

Teachings are open only to twice born men: those of top three *varnas* (castes)–brahmins (priests), *kshatriyas* (warriors and rulers) and *vaishyas* (merchants and land owners). *Shudras* (serfs) and women are denied teachings.

Karma becomes a notion of fulfiling one's personal duty (*svadharma*) depending on one's caste.

Brahmin status is eventually given to temple priests of the non-orthodox traditions (see next page).

Continues on the next page

Classical Yoga (*Yoga Sutra*): placed around the 2nd century CE, but not in the form we have today. An eightfold system which draws on yogic meditation practice and displays Buddhist influences. It has similar views to Samkhya philosophy, but has a notion about *ishvara* (the Lord). No original commentary exists: earliest are written from a Samkhya perspective.

Samkhya: Systemised by Ishvara Krishna (5th century CE). It has pluralistic ideas of many spirits (*purushas*), but no God. A possible psychological and metaphysical view, which aims to bridge the gap between religion and philosophy. Some notions are also found in the *Katha Upanishad*.

Vedanta (2-3rd century CE): Claims to be an interpretation of the *Vedas*, but concentrates mainly on the *Upanishads*. Draws on various ideas, such as Buddhism and is paired with Mimasa philosophy. It is not an isolated, static system. The influential *Brahma Sutra* is written around 400CE and attempts to explain the *Upanishads*, but does not satisfactorily resolve the idea of the world evolving out of Brahman into a purely monistic system.

Advaita Vedanta: Shankara (788-820 CE) introduces 'misperceptions' (*maya*), which support his ideas on non-dualism. He writes a commentary on the *Brahma Sutra*, which has a huge impact and then concentrates mainly on the *Upanishads*. He is also credited with a commentary on the *Bhagavad Gita* and with forming various monastic orders, but little is known about his life overall.

Ramanuja (11th century CE) drew on the devotion of Vishnu in the South of India and is the founder of Sri Vaisnavism. His teachings are often termed 'qualified non-dualism'. The world is not an illusion and seen as Vishnu's body. He wrote commentaries on the *Brahma Sutra* and the *Bhagavad Gita*.

173

ELEMENTS OF HINDUISM
(continued from the previous page)

PERIOD 4+
Devotional Developments

It is worth noting that around the beginning of the common era there was a growing trend in stupa worship in the Buddhist tradition and the mention of 'houses of God' (early temple structures) in the Hindu spiritual tradition. Interestingly, Mahayana Buddhism also brings in a notion of grace.

Bhakti (devotion) can be seen as a reaction of the ordinary people to more rigid orthodox beliefs and practices. In India it draws on the Vishnu, Krishna and Shiva mythology. There is emphasis on following a guru and is caste inclusive. Liberation is open to all and the notion of grace comes in as an essential aspect.

The Epics are compiled: the *Mahabharata* (which is made up of various stories woven together) and the *Ramayana* (which is based upon an incarnation of Vishnu in the form of Rama).

The *Bhagavad Gita* (some place as late as 2nd century CE) is placed as part of the *Mahabharata*. It discusses ideas popular at the time (asceticism, Buddhist and Jain beliefs and practices, the *Vedas*, *Upanishads* and various yoga exercises) and comes up with its own synthesis: a particular type of *bhakti* (loyalty and devotion to Krishna while acting in the world). Because of its popularity, it also became influential in the more orthodox sections of the Hindu tradition.

In the 6th century CE in the South of India, *bhakti* develops into a creative form with devotional acts and poetry being written. Before this period there was a growing trend in what are termed 'sants': a wide term that is used to describe a specific group of wondering poet-saints. The Buddha referred to them, so were there before 500 BCE as an undercurrent.

Sophisticated literature emerges in the North of India and the people are invited to the South to spreads their ideas. There is construction of many temples, largely dedicated to Shiva or Vishnu. The custom of going on a pilgrimage starts and there is a growing emphasis on symbolic erotic art used in temple structures.

The *Srimad Bhagavatam* is written around the 10th century CE, but some say it is much older. The author is aware of a text from around the 5th century CE, known as the *Vishnu Purana*, but adds to and expands the Krishna mythology. It is a direct influence of the bhakti poets. The *Srimad Bhagavatam* triggers a massive devotional movement in the North.

Tantric texts (*agamas*) are produced as early as the 4th century CE and placed emphasis on the Goddess and her Creative Power.

In the 10th century CE, devotional poets, such as Nayanas and Alvars, influenced a growing devotional movement in the South of India. Important figures in this movement are Basavanna (1106-1167) and Chaitanya (1485-1536).

SRI AUROBINDO'S MODEL OF THE SELF

Sachchidananda
(*Sat-Chit-Ananda*)
The One Divine Being with a triple aspect of pure Existence, Consciousness and Bliss.

Supermind/Supramental
The Truth Consciousness, the Highest Divine Consciousness and Force in the universe.

Overmind
The overmind draws down Truths separately and gives them separate identities.

Intuition
What is thought-knowledge in the higher mind becomes illumination and direct intimate vision.

Illumined Mind
A mind no longer of higher thought, but of spiritual light.

Higher Mind
A luminous thought-mind whose instrumentation is through elevated thought-power and comprehensive mental vision. Here one begins to become aware of the true Self.

Ordinary Mind
Linked with cognitive intelligence, perceptions and reactions and has 3 aspects:

  Mind Proper
  Thinking, intellect, realisation and expression of ideas.

  Vital Mind
  Impulses, emotions and sensations that seek fulfilment and enjoyment. Dynamic will and action, occupied with movement for its own sake.

  Physical Mind
  Concerned with physical things; limited by a physical view and experience of things.

Subconscient
(the subconscious)
Includes a large part of the physical mind, vital being and body consciousness.

Inconscient
(the unconscious)
All powers above ordinary consciousness progressively evolve and emerge out of the inconscient. The first emergence of being is matter.

APPENDIX II
The Siddhis and Christian Wisdom

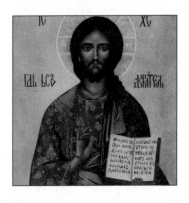

*Jesus showed a way of living and acting in the world
with compassionate understanding.
Through his teachings, spread hope, spiritual light
and knowledge of a life eternal.*
SWAMI DHARMANANDA

*Teachings of unity, equality, peace, forgiveness,
unconditional love, universal wisdom and leading by example
are the signs of the great masters of spirituality.*
SANTOSHAN

How can we fail to be struck by
the revealing growth around us of a strong mystical current,
actually nourished by the conviction that the universe,
viewed in its complete workings,
is ultimately lovable and loving?
PIERRE TEILHARD DE CHARDIN

God has gifted creation with everything necessary …
Humankind, full of all creative possibilities, is God's work.
Humankind is called to co-create …
HILDEGARD OF BINGEN

… the fruit of the Spirit is love, joy, peace, patience and kindness,
generosity, faithfulness, gentleness, and self-control.
GALATIANS

… to love God with all the heart, and with all the understanding,
and with all the strength, and to love one's neighbour as oneself
– this is much more important than all whole burnt offerings
and sacrifices.
GALATIANS

There is a river of creativity running through all things,
all relationships, all beings, all corners and centres of this universe.
We are here to join it, to get wet, to jump in,
to ride these rapids, wild and sacred as they be.
MATTHEW FOX

All of nature, its forms and
creatures are interrelated;
all will be returned to their
original source.
THE GOSPEL OF MARY MAGDALENE

The Miraculous Self

SANTOSHAN

There are different kinds of spiritual gifts,
but they all come from the same Spirit.
CORINTHIANS

There is a popular belief that the major world religions are against the use of psychic powers (termed *siddhis* in yogic wisdom) because they are obstacles to the spiritual life. Contrary to this idea, the beginnings of many global spiritual traditions invariably have a founder or early leader displaying supernormal gifts, and in the course of a religion's growth one will invariably find holy men and women with various psychic abilities.

Ancient scriptures often mention a variety of phenomena that can include the hearing of voices, seeing of visions, reading other people's minds and the ability to levitate. Today one hears of mystics from different traditions performing miracles, such as healings, materialising objects, or Tibetan Buddhists who consult oracles who are said to enter into trance states and have deities speak through them in order to offer spiritual guidance and make predictions.

In opposition to these practices, we find the Buddha condemning the use of psychic powers in the *Kevaddha Sutta* and individuals, such as the 20th Century yogi Gopi Krishna, claiming that the great modern Indian saints never endorsed the exhibition of psychic gifts or the working of miracles. To clarify some points on this subject, the following pages include views from influential teachings found in the Christian tradition and comparisons with Buddhism and Hindu yoga.

The first book I wrote with Glyn Edwards, *Tune in to your Spiritual Potential*, is worth referring to on this, in the chapter on psychic powers, which considers whether some abilities should be classed as supernatural, spiritual, or not. The points made in the chapter would distract from the main focus of this appendix and in order to cut down on repetition the words supernatural, supernormal and miraculous have been adopted.

Supernormal powers in Christianity

Similar to Jesus, St. Paul is presented in the New Testament as being a great miracle worker and is credited with the gift of healing. Paul's letters show that various psychic and miraculous gifts were part of early Christianity. He gave detailed instruction about the use of miraculous powers, prophecy, healing and speaking in tongues. However, he warns that if one has such gifts, but does not have love, one has nothing. Later on the practice of speaking in tongues was seen as heretical by the established church. Even today the Catholic Church considers it as an indication of diabolical intervention.

Visions and various phenomena persistently appear in the lives of the Christian mystics. St. Teresa of Avila is said to have levitated and had visions of angels. The stigmatists Padre Pio and Theresa Neuman are both reported to have had the ability of healing, bilocation and to have performed various other miracles. Sometimes people witnessed a perfume emanating from Padre Pio, especially the odour of violets, lilies, roses and incense. It was seen as a sign that God had bestowed some grace on those who noticed it.

What comes over in the lives of Catholic mystics is that they do not seek to attain supernatural gifts. Nor do they encourage others to possess them, as they are seen as a Divine blessing, given by God. St. Teresa advises beginners that it is best to resist them, believing the soul will advance quicker for doing so. The emphasis is on the practice of contemplation, prayer and moral conduct.

Nonetheless, although it appears that they do not seek the gifts, there are many accounts of them using them once they have manifested. St. Teresa's spiritual life and career as an abbess was governed by the voices she heard. The voices even warned her of coming events. St. John of the Cross wrote that people should not rejoice in the possession of the gifts, but rejoice in the benefit of being able to serve God through them.

But St. John warned that the gifts can be used wrongly to deceive people and believed that there were some that were true and some that were not. Catholic mystics appear unanimous in warning against the danger of attributing too much importance to them.

On the subject of visions – whether objective or subjective – author Albert Farges pointed out the importance of examining them for clearness and detail: to distinguish between that which comes from nature, from God, from the imagination or the devil; although most liberal minded Christians would not believe in the devil these days. Farges believed that such visions should appear spontaneously without preparation and disappear in the same manner.

He mentions two types of visions, clear and obscure, the obscure being beyond ordinary imagery and ties in with other traditions where the mystic is often lost for words to describe something beyond everyday experience.

For the Catholic mystic, supernormal visions and voices can be seen as a stage which may happen. But there are other stages where what is sometimes called the mystic death or dark night of the soul occurs, where one is not always aware of any voice or vision.

The renowned writer on Christian mysticism Evelyn Underhill believed that mystical visions and voices had a life enhancing quality, and were the means through which the seeing self truly approached God. In other words they are not only necessary phenomena for seeking union with God, but important experiences that bring about positive changes in an individual's spiritual growth.

A comparison with Hindu and Buddhist wisdom

On the one hand Catholic mystics do not aim to attain these gifts, as they must be given by God. On the other, St. Paul advocates the desire for spiritual gifts, especially prophecy.

In comparison, the superknowledges (psychic powers) in Buddhism and the *siddhis* in the *Yoga Sutra* are attained through one's own efforts. They involve bending one's mind to the realm of wondrous gifts, becoming invisible and multiple forms, penetrating solid matter, levitating, gaining clairaudience and clairvoyant insight in order to see into the hearts of others, as well as into one's previous lives and seeing

179

how creatures pass from one state of being to another.

Although many of these gifts might be interpreted as being internal meditative states rather than outward displays of supernatural power, they are an essential part of the teachings. They are aimed for in order to help overcome the effects of karma and attain liberation. They do not imply that the practitioner has reached a true state of sanctity. It is the realisation that all inhibiting qualities have been overcome that is important, as this guarantees deliverance from the influence of karmic performing actions that bind one to the realm of unsatisfactory living and conditioned existence.

A popular opinion aired by some advocates of non-dualistic Vedanta philosophy is that Patanjali's *Yoga Sutra* recommends giving up psychic powers. This opinion has arisen through a belief in the world being an illusion and, therefore, anything belonging to it – including psychic powers – has little value. This is in fact a misleading interpretation and has created some uninformed prejudice in some circles. The respected yoga practitioner and scholar Georg Feuerstein pointed out in his commentary to the work, that the belief in psychic abilities not being part of Patanjali's teachings on Self-realisation is demonstrably wrong, as they cannot be separated from the essential organic and unitary structure of yoga.

According to the *Bhagavata Purana*, although the gifts are seen as being given by God, they are also viewed as being partly earned through one's efforts, as one has to deliberately meditate on a feature of God to have them bestowed upon oneself. But it should be noted that the powers are not for the attainment of mastery over the elements, but for mastery over one's self. All yogic traditions make this point. However, the belief that various traditions avoid using the powers for fear of becoming overpowered or distracted by them, or because they are a block to spiritual growth, goes against the evidence. It is clear that once attained the powers are frequently used.

Christian mystics believe that they can be used to serve God. Brahmin priests use their power and chant mantras and recite prayers to maintain cosmic order. The Buddha sometimes used them for conversion – even though he would have normally converted by preaching – and on the nights of his enlightenment. He was well aware that the practice of meditation led to the possession of psychic gifts.

What the Buddha primarily objected to was the unnecessary display of psychic powers. For instance, in the early monastic rules there is a story about the Buddha rebuking one of the monks for displaying supernatural powers merely to impress people. Falsely claiming possession of miraculous gifts is one of only four offences which can lead to expulsion from the monastic community, which shows how serious early Buddhists were about such things.

The powers are seen as possible signs that a monk has suspended the laws of nature and overcome binding influences. But one has to be careful not to be tempted too much by them and so lose sight of the ultimate goal of liberation from birth, death and rebirth.

The essentials of spirituality

Maybe the reason for some being against their use is that they want to encourage people to focus more on spiritual living than on psychic phenomena. But even here there is a problem, as the powers are used to help people become enlightened or to serve God and so become more spiritual forces for good in the world.

There is also a problem for those who have naturally manifested such abilities. Are they meant to suppress them? This could cause psychological problems. If a gift has naturally arisen, surely it would be better to understand something about it and use it selflessly and wisely.

Where all traditions seem to agree is in the warning that these abilities should not be desired for their own sake, or as a means for egotistical display or self-promotion. The emphasis is often on practices such as humility, non-attachment, skilful actions – thought, word and deed – or devotion to God.

It ought to be mentioned that to be classed as a mystic, one need not display any miraculous powers other than qualities of compassion, wisdom and living virtuously. All one needs to live a spiritual life is to practise self-mastery and transform one's overall nature into good. The display of psychic or miraculous powers in itself does not necessarily indicate an enlightened being.

In a documentary series made for English television, Bede Griffiths mentioned how Catholicism had mistakenly viewed supernormal powers as being either from God or from the devil, whereas in India the distinction between the psychic and the spiritual had been more accurately understood. "In India", he pointed out, "they have recognised that there is a vast psychic realm, which is neither good nor bad; it is ambivalent."

I think it is essential to bear Father Bede's observations in mind and to realise that it is how the gifts are used and influence one's life and conduct that determines their worth.

It should be noted that what might be classed as an extrasensory faculty by some might be seen as a miraculous gift by others. We also need to bear in mind that any practice, such as prayer or meditation, which is believed to have an effect, is a belief in psychic or miraculous power. Even if there is a psychological explanation for what is happening. If an individual holds a belief in a power that brings about a change, then it implies a belief in some kind of supernormal force. Visualisation practices can, for instance, be viewed as a way of entering into and working with the psychic level of our being. In fact, nothing can be known unless it first appears – in some form or another – as a psychic impression.

Whatever conclusion one wishes to make, it is clear that psychic or miraculous gifts, although not essential to the spiritual and mystical life, are intrinsically bound-up with and are frequently by-products of it. It is only when one does not heed the warning about attachment to them and uses them for self-promotion that they become obstacles to the path.

APPENDIX III
Buddhist Wisdom

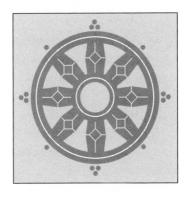

May we all proceed in knowledge,
wisdom and understanding.
SWAMI DHARMANANDA

There is potential for growth in every moment
if we are prepared to awaken to it.
SANTOSHAN

To shun all evil. To do good. To purify the heart.
This is the teaching of the Buddhas.
THE DHAMMAPADA

In the gap between thoughts, nonconceptual wisdom shines continuously.
MILAREPA

The aim of Zen is the breaking-up of the dualistic structure
of conscious-and-unconscious.
RICHARD DEMARTINO

One Nature, perfect and pervading, circulates in all natures,
One Reality, all-comprehensive, contains within itself all realities.
The one Moon reflects itself wherever there is a sheet of water,
and all the moons in the waters are embraced within the one moon.
The Dharma-body of all the Buddhas enters into my own being.
And my own being is found in union with theirs …
The Inner light is beyond praise and blame.
Like space it knows no boundaries, yet it is even here, within us,
ever retaining its serenity and fullness.
YUNG-CHIA TA-SHIH

Truly, the wise do not pretend,
For they have understood the way of the world.
By final knowledge the wise are quenched:
They have crossed over attachment to the world.
DEVATASAMYUTTA

A Selfless Path

SANTOSHAN

Be a light unto thyself.
THE BUDDHA

Similar to various paths of yoga, the Buddha's teachings encompass the cultivation of ethical conduct, self-exploration and overcoming the split between subject and object experience.

The early teachings are about personal effort and responsibility, and realising that the path to spiritual enlightenment lies within us. We are the ones who are in charge of our unfoldment and need to discover what steps can be taken to achieve freedom from the entanglements of life and the many forms of discontentment. To begin we must start from where we are and find methods for bringing about changes in the way we think, feel and act and perceive life.

The path the Buddha recommends for doing this is a therapeutic one that leads to deep intuitive insight and seeing things in their true nature. When this is achieved we no longer see life as made-up of separate phenomena and become awakened to the interrelatedness of all existence. By following the eightfold path we are able to transform our overall understanding and manifest unconditional compassion.

A noble silence

Because the Buddha believed it was impossible to describe Nirvana to those who had not experienced it, he frequently observed a noble silence on questions about it. It would be like trying to describe colour, shape and form to someone who had been blind from birth.

The Buddha believed it would not help to describe what could not be understood until it had been realised for oneself. It would confuse people with concepts, which would imprison the mystery and not help them discover the Truth for themselves. What was more important than entering into discussion about Nirvana was to find a way of overcoming the problems of worldly existence.

To illustrate this point, there is a story in the early teachings about a man who had been shot with an arrow, which describes how there would be no point in his asking questions about what weapon it was propelled from, whether it was a long-bow or crossbow, what string had been used and so on. What would be of more value would be to have the arrow removed so as to stop the man's suffering. This is a pragmatic approach which encourages us to attend to what is more important first. Our houses are on fire with anger, desires and misconceptions. We have enough work on our hands in putting out these fires – questions about the Ultimate will have to wait!

There is common sense to the Buddha's approach. People can use intellectual concepts as a distraction, instead of getting down to doing some practical work that relates and is more helpful to the here and now of everyday life and spirituality. Intellectual pursuits can be used as a way of burying our heads in the sand, instead of finding ways and means to live a balanced and wholesome life.

Unsatisfactoriness

The essential teachings of the Buddha can be unpacked from his Four Noble Truths. They are often compared with steps towards the cure of an illness:

(1) Diagnosis of the illness.
(2) Identification of the conditions that caused the illness.
(3) The prognosis, which is good, as it indicates that there is a way to a complete recovery.
(4) Steps to be taken to cure the illness: the Buddha's Eightfold Path.

The first noble truth (opposite) is an observation about the human condition and existence of *duhkha* (unsatisfactoriness). The word *'duhkha'* is often translated as 'suffering', which has led some to believe that the Buddha's teachings are a negative path to enlightenment. But

Three marks of existence
All conditioned things constantly change and are impermanent.
All conditioned things are unsatisfactory.
All things are selfless.

The Four Noble Truths
1. The human condition is characterised by unsatisfactoriness.
2. The cause of unsatisfactoriness is desire.
3. Unsatisfactoriness can be overcome.
4. The way to overcome unsatisfactoriness – the Noble Eightfold Path.

The Eightfold Path
1. Right view.
2. Right intention.
3. Right speech.
4. Right action.
5. Right livelihood.
6. Right effort.
7. Right mindfulness.
8. Right concentration.

Three fires that have to be put out
Desire, anger, and the lack of understanding and insight (ignorance).

Five precepts
To abstain from taking life (harmlessness).
To abstain from taking what is not given.
To abstain from sexual misconduct.
To abstain from false speech.
To abstain from intoxicants which cloud the mind.

Four sublime states
Extending unlimited, universal love and good-will to all living beings.
Compassion for all beings who are suffering, in trouble and afflicted.
Sympathetic joy in other people's success, welfare and happiness.
Equanimity in all circumstances of life.

we should realise that the Buddha was being a realist – particularly if we think of what life must have been like in his time: disease, tribal disputes and a short life expectancy would have been common then.

However, 'unsatisfactoriness' is seen as a more accurate word for *duhkha* and helpful translation for understanding the Buddha's teachings. Studies by scholars of early Buddhism confirm this. The Buddha did not deny that happiness could be found in the world, but pointed out that it would not last. His teachings aim to help us find lasting contentment, to cultivate loving-kindness, and to discover freedom from hatred and unskilful states of mind.

Pursuit of worldly pleasure is seen by the Buddha to go hand-in-hand with unsatisfactoriness due to all conditioned things being impermanent. The Buddha's teachings on conditioned existence are about everything being caused by numerous other factors. Death is preceded by birth and life, rebirth is determined by karmic actions. When one thing happens it causes something else to happen and so on. The way we perceive life is created by and is the outcome of various influences. All things come into being and pass away and are dependent on other things for their existence.

It is because we have not realised and accepted conditioned life, and that all things are impermanent and constantly undergoing change, that we encounter unsatisfactoriness. On a basic level we might gain enjoyment by partying all night. But the next morning we would no doubt feel tired, stiff and have a hang-over. Even if we continuously did what we enjoy most, we would still encounter unsatisfactoriness, as there would be times when events would not go the way we had planned. We may also have days when we feel under the weather or bored with the repetition of doing the same activity.

The prime cause of unsatisfactoriness is desire and a lack of knowledge about the way things really are. Desires are not just about wanting things that we have not got, but also about longing for life to remain the same and for any unpleasantness to be taken away.

This process of yearning for things to remain the same can be seen as happening at various levels, including the realms of thought, feelings and sensory enjoyment. We can see how consistency gives us a sense of security and order. We are after all creatures of habit and want our health to be good, our jobs to be safe, our emotions to be stable, the trains and buses to run on time, a quiet home that always keeps the rain out and warms us in the winter, and to have good and lasting relationships with our friends and family. Yet it can be seen that it is this expectation that causes us frustration, discontent and unsatisfactoriness.

For the Buddha, overcoming this problem lay in cultivating a realistic view, one which encompasses an acceptance of things as they come into being and pass away, and an awareness of what it is that causes us to see life in a certain way. We have to change our overall understanding, so that we no longer see ourselves as separate individuals with self-centred desires that conflict with how life truly is. Through putting the Buddha's key practices of right view, right effort and right mindfulness into action, we can gain insight into how we psychologically work and ways to transform our overall selves and our daily encounters with discontentment.

Meditation

One of the Buddha's key practices is meditation. Comparing the Buddha's teachings on meditation with the *Yoga Sutra's* eightfold path there are some subtle differences. The practice of *pratyahara* (sensual withdrawal) is not specifically mentioned by the Buddha, but it can be seen to tie in with one of his four absorption states. The breath is not held, as in *pranayama* practices, and self-study, with its links with mindfulness and therapeutic analysis, is promoted more clearly as something to be performed in all areas and activities of life.

But we are not comparing eggs with eggs here. The *Yoga Sutra* is a potted summary of practices, whereas the Pali Cannon includes a vast and detailed collection of the Buddha's teachings.

As in the *Yoga Sutra* (which displays some Buddhist influences), the Buddha's meditative path includes moral conduct as an initial and ongoing stage, then the cultivation of a positive outlook and an awareness of one's thoughts, words and deeds for the purpose of eliminating any inhibiting patterns. Finally, all of life's experience – body, mind, feelings and external phenomena – is reflected upon as transient and being in a continual state of change. This leads to an increased clarity and focusing of the mind, which brings about an awakening to wider states of consciousness.

The word Buddha means 'enlightened' or 'awake', implying someone who has woken-up to seeing things clearly. Through both meditation and awareness we objectively observe life internally and externally, and transform anything that stops us from seeing it realistically and dualistically – overcoming the split between inner and outer existence. We become more mindful and conduct ourselves in a fully conscious way, even when engaged in activity. Life becomes concentrated on the present moment, instead of being wrapped-up in problems of the past or anxieties about, or predominantly self-centred desires for, the future.

Right effort is particularly important as it is the willing/ volitional factor that motivates us to do the work that is necessary for transforming unskilful states of mind, and for cultivating positive qualities and insight into the truth of the Buddha's teachings.

Interconnectedness

We must realise that what is fed into the unconscious will affect our conscious awareness. It is because of our past conditioning that we see ourselves as physically unconnected with exterior life. Our senses create the appearance of our being singular and distinctly separate from other people and objects around us and in the universe.

Yet not only did the Buddha tell us that this is a wrong perception, but also quantum physicists have now discovered this to be true. On a sub-atomic level there is no clear boundary between different forms of life, objects and phenomenon. Similarly the research of Rupert Sheldrake into morphogenic fields and resonance also shows an interconnectedness in nature, of which we ourselves are a part of.

Five aspects of ourselves

The Buddha identified five aspects of our human nature, known as *skandhas* (constituents):

(1) Body.
(2) Feelings.
(3) Conceptual abilities.
(4) Volitional activities.
(5) Consciousness.

Collectively the *skandhas* can be seen to make-up the fundamental basics of our individuality. The key to why we see ourselves as separate beings lies with number three: the identifying and conceptualising part of ourselves.

There are at least three ways of looking at the *skandhas*. One is that they partly explain the Theravadin Buddhist doctrine of 'no self'. The second, which ties in with the other two, is that the self that is being referred to is only the ego-self – not the higher Self of the Hindu yogic tradition. The third is that they give us a psychological model of how we work and perceive ourselves as separate personalities.

The latter does not signify that there is no self and links with other teachings of the Buddha, which relate to the human condition and looks for ways in which we can be helped, i.e. that by understanding different aspects of ourselves and how we function, we can change the way we view life and overcome unsatisfactoriness. We should remember that the Buddha never said that we do not exist. The idea of no self is in fact one of six false views that he mentioned. What he was trying to say was that there is no self that is totally independent and separate from other life and influences for it to exist.

Some Buddhists believe that because there cannot be found an individual unchanging essence which can be called an 'I', this implies that there is no self. This includes the yogic understanding of the *atman* – the idea of a self merely being the collective name for the sum of the parts. But as mentioned before, speculation on anything other than what the Buddha saw as necessary to become liberated from unsatisfactoriness was not encouraged by him.

To say there is 'a self' or 'no self' – particularly an eternal spiritual Self – is to enter into metaphysical speculation, which the Buddha believed would only confuse us with concepts that would get in the way of realising Nirvana for ourselves and distract us from what was more important.

In the early Pali teachings the Buddha claimed to be neither an eternalist nor a nihilist, which puts him slightly at odds with Upanishadic wisdom and Mahayana understanding about our eternal Buddha nature; though such a stance doesn't completely rule them out. In fact the Buddha accepted that beneficial teachings could be included as part of the *dharma* (the teachings), which demonstrates how open minded and inclusive he was.

His approach is really 'non-theistic'. To say his path is or isn't about God would equally miss the point of what he was teaching. His interests lie in how we experience life, rather than asking theological questions about how we got here or where we will go when we die.

Similarly, by building on the *Perfection of Wisdom Sutra's* teachings on emptiness, the influential Mahayana Buddhist philosopher Nagajuna also argued against conceptualism and metaphysical speculation, although even a non-conceptual philosophy can still be seen as just another concept.

Selflessness and karma

The Buddha's central message is about seeing things 'self-lessly'. By doing so, we overcome unsatisfactoriness, as we no longer have self-centred desires that would cause it. This also means that we can practise true compassion, as selflessness means seeing that we are not separate from others and their suffering. It is a cognitive change which leads to freedom and spiritual living. Any effort towards this goal will be of benefit because of the way in which it ties in with karma. In Buddhism, karma is about volitional activities, the intention behind the deed, which is the only one of the *skandhas* that produces karma, to either to our benefit or to our detriment. It is also bound up with ideas about desire, attachment, wrong thinking, unawareness and anger.

In following the steps of the Buddha's Eightfold Path and applying them, we begin to lead a more ethically responsible life. This is because when we truly see things as they are, we no longer act out of selfish motives, as we no longer over-identify with our individual self and its desires and attachments. Instead, we become desire-less and more impartial and begin to conduct ourselves with a pro-active attitude that works for the good of all.

In attaining this understanding we are no longer subject to habitual ways of thinking. Instead of reacting to life when things change beyond our control and don't go the way we expect them to, we accepts all things with equanimity and emanate loving-kindness to all.

Elements of Buddhism Chart

ELEMENTS OF BUDDHISM

The Buddha

❀ Siddhatta Gotama, who after his enlightenment became known as the Buddha, was born around the middle of the 6th century BCE in Lumbini, on the borders of present-day Nepal. He is said to have been a prince of the Shakya tribe and that is why he is sometimes referred to as Shakymuni Buddha (sage of the Shakya clan). He is considered to be only one in a long-line of Buddhas who incarnated before him.

❀ The Buddha's mother, Maya, died seven days after giving birth to him and a holy man predicted he would become either a great monarch or a spiritual teacher. He married and had a son who later became one of his followers. His father, Suddhodana, tried to protect him from the outside world and from becoming a holy man. But the Buddha saw three facts of life – old age, sickness and death – which made him question life and the continual cycle of death, rebirth and unsatisfactoriness. He also saw a fourth sight, a holy man, which led him to leave home and, together with five other adepts, to try various spiritual practices and teachings, including harsh asceticism. But he found that nothing fully helped him to change his overall being and so he began to look for a middle way between different extremes of living.

❀ In Bodhgaya he sat under a Bodhi tree and vowed to stay there until he became enlightened. Mara, a demon-like figure, tried to distract him and to tempt him with various desires. But the Buddha realised the truth of existence, saw the causes of all unsatisfactoriness, the influences of karma and previous actions and lives, and how these can be overcome.

❀ At first the Buddha thought these teachings would be too difficult for people to comprehend. But he then again met the five ascetics he had previously been with. After hearing the his first sermon on the 'Four Noble Truths' (called 'the first turning of the wheel of *dharma*') at the Deer Park in Sarnath, they became his first disciples.

❀ He formed a community (*sangha*) that was made up of monks, nuns and lay members, and subsequently became popular and influential in his own lifetime.

❀ He eventually died at Kusinagara at the age of eighty (his *paranirvana*) due to what appears to have been food poisoning. His teachings were remembered by various members of the monastic community and later recorded.

❁ His ashes were preserved as a relic inside a stupa at Kasinagara, which then became an important pilgrimage site for Buddhists. He is looked upon as a human being and respected as someone who has shown the way to living life freely and compassionately.

Key points about the teachings and Theravada Buddhism

❁ The first council meeting of monks and nuns was called soon after the Buddha's death in order to agree upon and remember the teachings. A century later, a second council was held. The teachings were not written down until after at least another century.

❁ The teachings are divided into three categories/baskets: (1) *Vinaya Pitaka*, basket containing rules for the monks and nuns, (2) *Sutta Pitaka*, basket containing the teachings of the Buddha, and (3) *Abhidamma Pitaka*, basket containing important psychological and philosophical commentaries, which attempt to systemise the Buddha's teachings. Although there is evidence that parts of the *Abhidamma Pitaka* were composed after the Buddha's death, the Theravada tradition maintains that the whole of its teaching can be traced back to the Buddha himself.

❁ Buddhism can be described as a 'non-theistic' religion. Although the Vedic gods still appear in the *Pali Canon* (the above collection of teachings), the Buddha focuses on the human condition and not on the existence of God. The Buddha remained silent on metaphysical speculation, as he saw it as unhelpful to discuss such matters.

❁ Someone who has attained Nirvana is someone who has blown out the three fires of desires, ignorance and anger, and is no longer bound to the cycle of birth, death and rebirth (*samsara*) and the unsatisfactoriness (*duhkha*) of life. Those who have become enlightened have woken up to seeing things as they are, i.e. as non-separate and without any essential lasting nature – everything being dependent on other conditions to bring it into being (termed 'dependent origination' in Buddhism).

❁ Dependent origination is a key concept in Buddhism. It is about the way different things cause other things to happen (many causes having many different effects) and is linked with how various parts of ourselves (the five *skandhas*: body, feelings, conceptual abilities, volitional activities and consciousness) create the appearance of a separate self.

ELEMENTS OF BUDDHISM

❀ The fundamental teachings of the Buddha are often referred to as 'the middle way', which is summarised in the Four Noble Truths and the Eight-fold Path.

❀ The Thee Jewels – 'I take refuge in the Buddha, the *dharma* and the *sangha*' – are like acknowledging a creed.

❀ Buddhism was initially an oral tradition that displayed a missionary activity from the start. It later spread through various trade routes into other countries which often adopted it for its pragmatic approach to life.

❀ The Buddha's teachings were influenced by notions of *samsara*, karma and liberation that were popular in India at the time. Liberation (Nirvana) was made open to everyone through self-effort.

❀ Karma is about the intentions behind one's deeds, and is also bound up with ideas about desire, attachment, wrong thinking, unawareness and anger. One cannot develop without undergoing the consequences of previous karma.

❀ The early commentaries list five categories of natural law, of which karma is connected with only one (No. 4): (1) changes in environment, such as the weather, (2) heredity, (3) workings of the mind, (4) human behaviour, and (5) the law governing the relationship and interdependence of all things.

❀ Buddhism's teachings are an ethical and psychological 'know thy self' system. The Buddha had his own insights and does not accept the *sruti* (revealed) teachings of the Hindu tradition.

❀ Early Buddhism rejected the use of the Sanskrit language and gave the teachings in local dialects, therefore making its wisdom available to all. However, Buddhists now use Sanskrit and Pali languages in countries that have no previous connections with these. It was not until the 19th century that the Pali Canon was mass-produced and made available to the public.

❀ Mind is seen as primarily pure, but becomes polluted by external impurities.

❀ For the Buddha, there is neither a 'self' nor 'no-self'. Theravada Buddhists later advocate a notion of 'no-Self' (*anatta*).

❀ Initially, compatible teachings could be seen as part of the Buddha's teachings (the *dharma*).

❀ One is allowed to interpret and apply the teachings oneself as an act of personal responsibility.

❀ Monks were told by the Buddha to spread 'the spirit of the teachings, but not the word'. *Abhidhamma* commentaries arguably changed this by being too specific and included notions about lots of *dharmas*, which are like atoms, and this may have been a contributory factor that caused Buddhism's great schism.

❀ Buddhism, like the *Upanishads*, is about transcending the ego and finding liberation in the Ultimate Reality. But both interpret this in different ways.

❀ Around the 3rd Century BCE the Buddhist monk Mahinda is credited with taking Buddhism from India to Sri Lanka, where it formed the last remaining school of early Buddhism – Theravada Buddhism – and spread to many other countries from there.

❀ It is said that there were eighteen early branches of Buddhism which arose because of disputes about the way the Three Jewels should be interpreted.

❀ Mahayana Buddhists, have in the past, sometimes unfairly called Theravada the 'lesser vehicle'. But Theravada Buddhists would never consider themselves to be following a less important path.

Mahayana Buddhism

❀ Mahayana Buddhism was formed between the 1st century BCE and the 1st century CE. Arguably, it highlighted much of what was partly or already there, such as the *bodhisattva* ideal, all things being selfless ('empty' in Mahayana Buddhism), compassion, wisdom and skill in means.

❀ The Buddha is semi-deified by Mahayana Buddhists, and they incorporate idea about there being 'three Buddha bodies': the earthly body in which all Buddhas appear to help liberate all beings (body of transformation); the body of the Buddha in a heavenly Buddha-realm where beings enjoy the truth they embody (body of delight); and the nature of the Buddha which is identical with the fundamental essence of the universe and the Ultimate Transcendental Reality (body of great order). The latter also includes the teachings of the Buddha.

❀ Mahayana Buddhists developed the idea of a perfect 'Buddha nature' that everyone possesses, which means that all people have the capacity to become a Buddha and exhibit wisdom and compassion.

❀ The Buddha is said to have given the teachings of Mahayana Buddhism on a rock at Vultures' Peak, and these are seen by Mahayanists as being higher teachings that all previous schools of Buddhism were not ready to receive. But they also incorporate the early teachings.

❀ Within Mahayana Buddhism there are two main philosophical systems: Madhyamaka and Yogacara. The latter is also called the Mind Only School and was founded by Asanga in the 4th century CE. It introduces the concept of 'store consciousness' (*alaya-vijnana*). These two schools present different interpretations of the *Perfection of Wisdom Sutra*. It has been suggested that their two most important philosophers, Nagarjuna (150-250 CE) the founder of the Madhyamaka school, and Vasubhandu (4/5th century CE) the founder of the Yogacara school, are not necessarily trying to introduce a new vision, but are attempting to reaffirm the original teachings of the Buddha. There is an ongoing debate as to whether or not Yogacara is an idealist system that looks upon everything as a product of the mind and consciousness.

❀ Tantra/Vajrayana Buddhism comes out of the Mahayana tradition and develops a third strand of Buddhism.

❀ In Mahayana Buddhism, the use of Sanskrit, the notion of grace, and the practice of devotion became strongly part of the tradition.

❀ Large monasteries with scholarly libraries were built in Bihar in India. Nalanda University being perhaps the largest centre for Buddhist studies that the world has ever known.

❀ Buddhism is believed to have been in decline in India by the time of the Muslim invasion, and from the 12th century CE it disappeared almost completely in India.

Becoming a worldwide tradition

❀ At a popular level Buddhism can often be about gaining merit for one's self and one's ancestors in order to achieve advantages in one's present life or a favourable rebirth. This can be done by chanting, lighting incense in front of statues, or making offerings – flowers, food, clothes or money – to a local monastery or temple. Monks may hold a special service for a departed relative in order for him or her to gain merit.

ELEMENTS OF BUDDHISM

✿ The various Buddhist traditions were kept alive by their spreading to other countries, such as Thailand, Burma, Cambodia, China, Japan, Korea, Vietnam, Sri Lanka and Tibet. Buddhism originally spread to China through central Asia around the beginning of the modern era and made its way into other Eastern countries from there. In China it became influenced by some Taoist ideas and Confucian ethics, and evolved into two main schools: Pure Land and Chan Buddhism (the latter is known as Zen in Japan, Son in Korea and Thien in Vietnam). Initially Buddhist monks were seen as parasitic in China and suffered persecution. Eventually, however, they became self-sufficient, instead of relying on offerings from the lay community, which helped to make them more acceptable there.

✿ Other influential branches of Mahayana Buddhism have surfaced in countries such as Japan and Vietnam. In Tibetan Buddhism there are some elements of the local Bon religion mixed with it.

✿ Now Buddhism is also very much a Western tradition with people presented with a choice of practices, such as Theravada, Tibetan, Chan, Nichiren Buddhism, etc., and there are many Western converts in America, Europe and Australia. Some Westerners now live in families having had at least three generations of Buddhists. Various forms of Buddhism have adapted to the needs of Western students. Many have promoted unity with other faiths and have looked for a common human core, as seen in the teachings and practices of Thich Nhat Hanh at Plum Village in France and the talks and books of the Dalai Lama. Popular writers, such as Jack Kornfield, have highlighted Buddhism's psychotherapeutic values. Technically, like Hindu yoga, we can no longer speak of it as being just an Eastern tradition. There is also a growing healthy interest in 'Engaged Buddhism', which focuses on practical social activism and aims to bring about positive changes in some countries and communities.

Bibliography

Adiswarananda, Swami, *Meditation and its Practices: A Definitive Guide to Techniques and Traditions of Meditation in Yoga and Vedanta*, Skylight Paths, Woodstock, 2003.

Almass, A. H., *Spacecruiser Inquiry: True Guidance for the Inner Journey*, Shambhala, Boston and London, 2002.

Amaldas, Swami, *Christian Yogic Meditation (Ways of Prayer – No. 8)*, Dominican Publications, Dublin, 1983.

Ambikananda Saraswati, Swami (translated by), *The Uddhava Gita: The Final Teachings of Krishna*, Frances Lincoln, New Delhi, 2000.

Assagioli, Roberto, *Psychosynthesis: A Manual of Principles and Techniques,* Aquarian Press, California, 1993 (reprint).

Aurobindo, Sri, *A Conception of Supermind in the Veda*, article in the *All India Magazine*, February 2004, Aurobindo Society, Pondicherry.

————— , *Glossary of Terms in Sri Aurobindo's Writings,* Sri Aurobindo Ashram, Pondicherry, 1978.

————— , *A Greater Psychology: An Introduction to the Psychological Thought of Sri Aurobindo* (edited by A. S. Dalal), Tarcher/Putnam, New York, 2001.

————— , *The Integral Yoga: Sri Aurobindo's Teaching and Method of Practice* (compiled by Sri Aurobindo Ashram Archives and Research Library), Lotus Light, Twin Lakes, 2000 (2nd reprint).

————— , *Letters on Yoga: Part One,* Sri Aurobindo Ashram, Pondicherry, 1988 (5th reprint).

————— , *The Riddle of this World*, Sri Aurobindo Ashram, Pondicherry, 1997 (5th reprint).

————— , *The Synthesis of Yoga,* Sri Aurobindo Ashram, Pondicherry, 1988 (4th edition, 8th reprint).

————— , *Yoga – Its Meaning and Objects*, Sri Aurobindo Ashram, Pondicherry, (reprint from the *All India Magazine*, August 2002).

————— and the Mother, *An Introduction to True Spirituality: The Words of Sri Aurobindo and the Mother*, Sri Aurobindo Ashram, Pondicherry, (reprint from *All India Magazine*, November 1997).

Bhaskar, Roy, *Meta-Reality: The Philosophy of meta-Reality, Vol. 1, Creativity, Love and Freedom*, Sage, New Delhi, 2002.

Bodhi, Bhikku (translated by), *The Connected Discourses of the Buddha: A Translation of the Samyutta Nikaya*, Wisdom Publications, Boston, 2000.

Brockington, J. L., *The Sacred Thread*, Edinburgh University Press, Edinburgh, 1996 (2nd Edition).

Brunton, Paul, *The Secret Meaning Behind Yoga*, Weiser, York Beach, 1993 (reprint).

Burns, Douglas M., *Nirvana, Nihilism and Satori: The Wheel Publication No. 117-119*, Buddhist Publication Society, Kandy, Sri Lanka, 1983 (2nd reprint).

Callahan, Sara, *Why the Buddha did not Answer the so-called 'Unanswered Questions'* (unpublished essay), London, February 1998.

Carty, Rev. Charles Mortimer, *Padre Pio: The Stigmatist*, Tan, Rockford (Illinois), 1973.

Chopra, Deepak, *Foreword* in *The Visionary Window: A Quantum Physicist's Guide to Enlightenment* by Amit Goswami, Quest Books, Wheaton, Illinois and Chennai (Madras), 2000.

Christie-Murray, David, *Voices from the Gods: Speaking in Tongues*, Routledge and Kegan Paul, London and Henley, 1978.

Cook, John, *The Book of Positive Quotations*, Fairview Press, Minneapolis, 1993.

Cope, Stephen, *Yoga and the Quest for the True Self*, Bantam, New York, 2000.

Craig, Edward (edited by), *The Shorter Routledge Encyclopedia of Philosophy*, Routledge, Abingdon, 2005.

Crowley, Vivianne, *Jungian Spirituality*, Thorsons, London, 1998.

Dharmananda Saraswati, Swami, *Breath of Life: Breathing for Health, Vitality and Meditation*, Dharma Yoga Centre, Harlow, 1996.

————— , *The Dynamic Body: Movements for Health, Vitality and Holistic Living*, Dharma Centre for Yoga, Spiritual Awareness and Healing, 2007 (pre-publication copy).

Dasgupta, Surendranath, *A History of Indian Philosophy: Vol. 1*, Motilal Banarsidass, Delhi, 1992 (reprint).

Edwards, Glyn and Santoshan, *Tune in to your Spiritual Potential*, Quantum, London, 1999.

————, *Unleash your Spiritual Power and Grow: Reflect and Learn to Trust the Power Within,* Quantum, London, 2007 (reprint).

Eliade, Mircea, *Yoga,* article in *The Encyclopedia of Religion: Vol. 15* (edited by Mircea Eliade), Macmillan, New York and London, 1987.

————, *Yoga: Immortality and Freedom,* Princeton University Press, New Jersey, 1990 (reprint).

Embrie, Ainslie T. (edited and revised by), *Sources of Indian Tradition: Vol. 1 – From the Beginning to 1800,* Columbia University Press, New York 1988.

Evans, Dylan, *Emotion: The Science of Sentiment,* Oxford University Press, Oxford, 2001.

Fadiman, James and Frager, Robert, *Essential Sufism,* Castle Book, Edison, New Jersey, 1997.

————, *Personality and Personal Growth,* Harper Collins, New York, 1994 (3rd edition).

Farges, Albert, *Mystical Phenomena: Compared with their Human and Diabolical Counterfeits,* Burns Oates and Washbourne, London, 1926.

Feuerstein, Georg, *The Deeper Dimensions of Yoga: Theory and Practice,* Shambhala, Boston and London, 2003.

————, *Encyclopedic Dictionary of Yoga,* Unwin, London 1990.

————, *Introduction to the Bhagavad Gita: Its Philosophy and Cultural Setting,* Quest Books, London, 1983 (1st Quest edition).

————, *The Philosophy of Classical Yoga,* Manchester University Press, Manchester, 1980.

————, *Textbook of Yoga: A Comprehensive Survey for the Western Student of the Schools, Literature, History, Philosophy & Practice of Yoga,* Rider and Company, London, 1975.

————, *Wholeness or Transcendence? Ancient Lessons for the Emerging Global Civilization,* Larson Publications, 1992 (revised and expanded edition).

————, *The Yoga-Sutras of Patanjali,* Inner Traditions International, Vermont, 1989 (reprint).

Fischer-Schreiber, Ingrid, Ehrhard, Franz-Karl, Friedrichs, Kurt and Diener, Michael S., *The Rider Encyclopedia of Eastern Philosophy and Religion,* Rider, London, 1989.

Forder, John and Forder, Eliza, *The Light Within: A Celebration of the Spiritual Path,* Usha Publications, Cumbria, 1995.

Freke, Timothy, *The Wisdom of the Hindu Gurus,* Godsfield Press, Alresford, Hants,

1998.

————, *The Wisdom of the Christian Mystics*, Godsfield Press, Alresford, Hants, 1998.

Fox, Matthew, *Creation Spirituality: Liberating Gifts for the Peoples of the Earth*, HarperSanFrancisco, 1990.

————, *Creativity: Where the Divine and the Human Meet*, Tarcher/Penguin, 2002.

————, *One River, Many Wells: Wisdom Springing from Global Faiths*, Gateway, 2000.

Gold, Victor Roland, Hoyt, JR., Thomas L., Ringe, Sharon H., Thistlewaite, Susan Brooks, Throckmorton, JR., Burton H., and Withers, Barbara A. (editors), *The New Testament and Psalms: An Inclusive Version*, Oxford University Press, Oxford and New York, 1995.

Goleman, Daniel (narrated by), *Destructive Emotions and How we can Overcome Them: A Dialogue with the Dalai Lama*, Bloomsbury, London, 2003.

Gollancz, Victor, *The New Year of Grace: An Anthology for Youth and Age*, Gollancz, London, 1964 (2nd reprint).

Gombrich, Richard F., *How Buddhism Began: The Conditioned Genesis of the Early Teachings*, Athlone, London and Atlantic Highland, 1996.

————, *Theravada Buddhism: A Social History from Ancient Benares to Modern Colombo*, Routledge, London, 1988.

Govindan, Marshall, *Kriya Yoga Sutra of Patanjali and the Siddhas: Translation, Commentary and Practice*, Kiya Yoga Publications, Quebec, 2000.

Gregory, Richard L. (edited by), *The Oxford Companion to the Mind*, Oxford University Press, Oxford, 1988 (reprint).

Griffiths, Bede, *Essential Writings* (selected with an introduction by Thomas Matus), Orbis Books, New York, 2004.

————, *The One Light: Bede Griffiths' Principal Writings* (edited with a commentary by Bruno Barnhart), Templegate, Springfield (Illinois), 2001.

Grof, Christina and Grof, Stanislav, *The Stormy Search for the Self: Understanding and Living with Spiritual Emergency*, Thorsons, London, 1991.

Guiley, Rosemary Ellen, *Harper's Encyclopedia of Mystical and Paranormal Experience*, Castle Books, Edison, 1991.

Gyeltsen, Geshe Tsultim, *Mirror of Wisdom: Teachings on Emptiness*, Thubten Dhargye Ling Publications, Long Beach, California, 2000.

Hamilton, Sue, *Anatta: A Different Approach*, adapted paper of a lecture given at the

School of Oriental and African Studies, London, Centre of South Asian Studies Seminar Series on 3rd November 1994.

Hardy, Friedhelm, *The Classical Religions of India*, Chapter 4 in *The World's Religions: The Religions of Asia* (edited by Friedhelm Hardy), Routledge, London, 1990 (reprint).

Heehs, Peter, *Sri Aurobindo: A Brief Biography*, Oxford University Press, New Delhi, 1999 (4th reprint).

Hopkins, Thomas J., *The Hindu Religious Tradition*, Wadsworth, California, 1971.

Iyengar, B. K. S., *Light on Life: The Journey to Wholeness, Inner Peace and Ultimate Freedom*, Rodale, London, 2005.

Jacobs, Alan (translated by), *The Gnostic Gospels: Including the Gospel of Thomas and the Gospel of Mary Magdalene*, Watkins Publishing, London, 2006.

———— (translated by), *The Principal Upanishads: A Poetic Translation*, O Books, Alresford, Hants, 2003.

Jayatilleke, K. N., *The Message of the Buddha*, George Allen and Unwin, London, 1975.

John of the Cross, St., (translated by Kavanaugh and Rodriguez), *The Collected Works of Saint John of the Cross (2nd revised edition)*, ICS, Washington, D.C., 1991.

Jung, C. G., *Memories, Dreams, Reflections*, Fontana press, 1983.

Keating, Thomas, *The Human Condition: Contemplation and Transformation* (with a foreword by Elaine Pagels), Paulist Press, New York and Mahwah, N.J., 1999.

King, Ursula, *Spirit of Fire: The Life and Vision of Teilhard de Chardin*, Orbis Books, New York, 1996 (5th printing).

Krishna, Gopi, *Higher Consciousness: The Evolutionary Thrust of Kundalini*, Julian Press, New York, 1994.

Lalita, *Choose Your Own Mantra*, Bantam Books, New York , 1978.

Lawless, Julia, and Allan, Judith, *Beyond Words: Dzogchen Made Simple*, Element, London, 2003.

Main, John, *Essential Writings* (selected with an introduction by Laurence Freeman), Orbis, New York, 2002.

Maitreya, The Ven. Balangoda Ananda (translation by), *The Dhammapada: The Path of Truth* (revised by Rose Kramer), Parallax Press, California, 1988.

Manjupuria, T. C., and Kumar (Majupuria), Rohit, *Gods and Goddesses: An Illustrated Account of Hindu, Buddhist, Tantric, Hybrid and Tibetan Deities*, Smt. M. D. Gupta, Lashkar, 1998.

Mascaro, Juan (translated by), *The Bhagavad Gita*, Penguin Books, Harmondsworth (Middlesex), 1962.

Mehta, Rohit, *From Mind to Super-Mind: A Commentary on the Bhagavad Gita*, Motilal Banarsidass, Delhi, 2000 (reprint).

Merton, Thomas, *Essential Writings* (selected with an introduction by Christine M. Bochen), Orbis, New York, 2002.

Mishra, Pankaj, *An End to Suffering: The Buddha in the World*, Picador, London, 2004.

Mukherjee, Jugal Kishore, *The Practice of Integral Yoga*, Sri Aurobindo Ashram, Pondicherry, 2003.

Muktibodhananda Saraswati, Swami (commentary by), *Hatha Yoga Pradipika*, Bihar School of Yoga, Munger, Bihar, 1993.

Nanamoli, Bhikkhu, *The Path of Purification: Visuddhimagga*, Buddhist Publication Society, Kandy, Sri Lanka, 1991 (5th Edition).

Nedumpalakunnel, George, *Realization of God according to Sri Aurobindo: A Study of a Neo-Hindu Vision on the Divinization of Man*, Claretian, Bangalore, 1979.

Nikhilananda, Swami (translated by), *The Bhagavad Gita*, Ramakrishna-Vivekananda Centre, New York, 1987 (5th reprint).

Nouwen, Henri J. M., *The Only Necessary Things: Living a Prayerful Life* (compiled and edited by Wendy Greer), Darton, Longman and Todd, London, 2002 (reprint).

Pandit, M. P., *Yoga in Savitri*, Dipti Publications, Pondicherry, 1995 (reprint).

————, *The Yoga of Self-Perfection: Talks Based on Sri Aurobindo's 'The Synthesis of Yoga'*, Dipti Publications, Sri Aurobindo Ashram, Pondicherry, 1983.

Payutto, P. A., *Good, Evil and Beyond*, Buddhadhamma Foundation, Bangkok, 1995 (2nd edition).

Prabhavananda, Swami (translated by), *Srimad Bhagavatam: The Wisdom of God*, Sri Ramakrishna Math, Mylapore, Madras, 1992 (reprint).

———— and Isherwood, Christopher (translation and commentary by), *How to Know God: The Yoga Aphorisms of Patanjali*, Vedanta Press, Southern California, 1981 (reprint).

———— (translated by), *Shankara's Crest-Jewel of Discrimination*, Vedanta Press, Hollywood, California, 1978 (reprint).

Olivelle, Patrick (translated by), *Upanishads*, Oxford University Press, Oxford and New York, 1996.

Radha, Swami Sivananda, *Kundalini Yoga*, Motilal Banarsidass, Delhi, 1992.

————, *Mantras: Words of Power,* Timeless Books, Spokane, 1994 (revised edition Radhakrishnan, S., *Indian Philosophy: Vol. 2,* Oxford University Press, Oxford, 1991 (4th reprint).

Rahula, Walpola, *What the Buddha Taught,* Gordon Frazer, London, 1978 (1st paperback edition).

————, *Zen and the Taming of the Bull,* Gordon Frazer, London, 1978.

Rama, Swami, Ballentine, Rudolph, and Ajaya, Swami, *Yoga and Psychotherapy: The Evolution of Consciousness,* The Himalayan Press, Honesdale, 1998 (10th reprint).

Ramachandra, T. (translated by), *Vedamritam: Immortal Vedic Hymns,* Sri Sanatam Dharma Trust (UK), London, 1981.

Rishabhchand, *The Integral Yoga of Sri Aurobindo,* printed at All India Press (no publisher credited), Pondicherry, 2000 (reprint).

Rukmani, T. S., *Siddhis in the Bhagavata Purana and in the Yoga-Sutras of Patanjali: A Comparison,* Chapter 16 in *Researches in Indian and Buddhist Philosophy: Essays in Honour of Prof. Alex Wayman* (edited by Ram Karan Sharma), Motilal Banarsidass, Delhi, 1993.

Sen, Indra, *Integral Psychology: The Psychological System of Sri Aurobindo,* Sri Aurobindo Ashram, Pondicherry, 1986.

Schumacher, E. F., *Small is Beautiful,* Harper & Row, New York, 1973.

Shastri, Hari Prasad, *Yoga,* Foyles, London, 1976 (reprint).

Sivananda, Swami, *The Practice of Yoga,* Divine Life Society, Himalayas, 1970.

————, *Raja Yoga: Life and Works of Swami Sivananda (Vol. 4),* Divine Life Society, Sivanandangar, 1986.

————, *The Science of Yoga: Japa Yoga (Vol. 12),* Yoga Vedanta Forest Academy, Rishikesh, 1971.

————, *The Science of Yoga: Pranayama (Vol. 7),* Yoga Vedanta Forest Academy, Rishikesh, 1971.

————, *Voice of the Himalayas,* Divine Life Society, Himalayas, 1996 (6th edition).

Smith, Curtis D., *Jung's Quest for Wholeness: A Religious and Historical Perspective,* SUNY, New York, 1990.

Staal, Frits, *Exploring Mysticism: A Methodological Approach,* University of California Press, California, 1975.

Story, Frances, *Kamma and Causality* and *Kamma and Freedom,* chapters in *Kamma and its Fruits* (edited by Nyanaponika Thera), Buddhist Publication Society,

Kandy, 1990 (2nd edition).

St Ruth, Diana and Richard, *Theravada Buddhism*, Global Books, Folkestone, Kent, 1998.

Suzuki, Shunryu, *Zen Mind, Beginner's Mind: Informal Talks on Zen Meditation and Practice*, Weatherhill, New York, 1995 (12th reprint).

Teilhard de Chardin, Pierre, *Pierre Teilhard de Chardin* (writings selected with an introduction by Ursula King), Orbis Books, New York, 1999.

Teresa, St., *The Life of Saint Teresa by Herself*, Penguin, London, 1959.

Thaker, Vimala, *Awakening to Total Revolution* (reprinted article in *What is Enlightenment?* magazine, September - December 2006, extracted from *Spirituality and Social Action: A Holistic Approach*, Berkley, California, 1984).

——— , *The Eloquence of Living: Meeting Life with Freshness, Fearlessness and Compassion*, New World Library, San Rafael, California, 1989.

Thera, Nyanaponika and Hecker, Hellmuth, (edited by Bhikkhu Bodhi), *Great Disciples of the Buddha*, Wisdom, Boston, 1997.

——— and Bodhi, Bhikkhu (translated and edited by), *Numerical Discourses of the Buddha: An Anthology of Suttas from the Anguttara Nikaya*, Altamira Press, Walnut Creek, Lanham, New York and Oxford, 1999.

Thich Nhat Hanh, *The Heart of the Buddha's Teachings: Transforming Suffering into Peace, Joy and Liberation*, Parallax Press, Berkeley (California), 1998.

Thittila, Maha Thera U., *The Fundamental Principles of Theravada Buddhism*, Chapter 2 in *The Path of the Buddha: Buddhism interpreted by Buddhists* (edited by Kenneth Morgan), Motilal Banarsidass, Delhi, 1993 (reprint).

Trainor, Kevin (general editor), *Buddhism*, Duncan Baird Publishers, London, 2004.

Trungpa, Chogyam, *The Collected Works of Chogyam Trungpa: Vol 3 – Cutting through Spiritual Materialism/The Myth of Freedom/The Heart of the Buddha/ Selected Writings*, Shambhala, Boston and London, 2003.

Underhill, Evelyn, *Mysticism: A Study in the Nature and Development in Man's Spiritual Consciousness (12th revised edition)*, Methuen and Co. Ltd., London, 1930.

Vrinte, Joseph, *The Quest for the Inner Man: Transpersonal Psychotherapy and Integral Sadhana*, Sri Mira Trust, Pondicherry, 1996.

Visser, Frank, *Ken Wilber: Thought as Passion,* State University of New York Press, Albany, 2003.

Vivekananda, *The Yogas and Other Works*, Ramkrishna-Vivekananda Centre, New York, 1984 (3rd reprint).

Vogl, Adalbert Albert, *Theresa Neumann: Mystic and Stigmatist, 1898-1962,* Tan Books, Rockford, Illinois, 1987.

Waida, Manabu, *Miracles,* article in *The Encyclopedia of Religion: Vol. 9* (edited by Mircea Eliade), Macmillan, New York and London, 1987.

Walshe, Maurice (translator), *The Long Discourses of the Buddha: A Translation of the Digha Nikaya,* Wisdom Publications, Massachusetts, 1995 (reprint).

Walsh, Roger and Vaughan, Frances (editors), *Paths Beyond Ego: The Transpersonal Vision,* Tarcher/Putnam, New York, 1993.

Warder, A. K., *Indian Buddhism,* Motilal Banarsidass, Delhi, 2000 (3rd revised edition).

Welwood, John, *The Journey of the Heart: The Path of Conscious Love,* HarperCollins, New York, 1990.

————— , *Towards a Psychology of Awakening: Buddhism, Psychotherapy and the Path of Personal and Spiritual Transformation,* Shambhala, Boston and London, 2000.

Weyer, Robert Van de (edited by), *366 Readings from Buddhism,* Arthur James, New Alresford, 2000.

Whicher, Ian, *The Integrity of the Yoga Darsana: A Reconsideration of Classical Yoga,* State University of New York Press, New York, 1998.

Wilber, Ken, *The Collected Works of Ken Wilber: Vol 2 – The Atman Project/Up from Eden,* Shambhala, Boston and London, 1999.

————— , *The Essential Ken Wilber: An Introductory Reader,* Shambhala, Boston and London, 1998.

Woodroffe, Sir John, *A Garland of Letters,* Ganesh and Co., Madras, 2001 (reprint).

————— , *The Serpent Power,* Ganesh and Co., Madras, 1992 (15th edition).

Woods, James Haughton , *The Yoga-System of Patanjali: Or the Ancient Hindu Doctrine of Concentration of Mind,* Motilal Banarsidass, Delhi, 1992 (reprint).

Yogananda, Paramahansa, *Autobiography of a Yogi,* Self-Realization Fellowship, Los Angeles (California), 1993 (12th edition).

————— (translation and commentary by), *God Talks with Arjuna: The Bhagavad Gita – Royal Science of God Realization,* Self-Realization Fellowship, Los Angeles (California), 1996 (2nd edition).

Yun, Ven. Master Hsing, *Buddhism and Psychology: Buddhism in Every Step (No. 14),* Buddha's Light Publishing, Hacienda Heights, 2004.

Zaehner, R. C. (translator), *Hindu Scriptures,* Everyman Library, London and New York, 1966 (reprint).

————— , *Hindu and Muslim Mysticism,* Oneworld, Oxford, 1994.

Glossary

Advaita (non-dualism) – the belief in there being ultimately only One Reality behind the many forms of life and matter in the universe (both seen and unseen).

Ahamkara (the 'I' maker) – the individual self or ego.

Ahimsa (non-harmfulness) – non-violence in thought, word or deed.

Ajna – the chakra that is seen as the seat of intuition, associated with the third-eye.

Akasha (ether/space) – the first of the five elements.

Ananda (bliss) – a condition of ultimate happiness experienced as part of the Ultimate Reality.

Antahkarana – the psyche or inner instrument through which we think, feel and discriminate. It consists of the lower mind (*manas*), the higher mind (*buddhi*) and the 'I' maker (*ahamkara*). The *Yoga Sutra* uses the term *chitta* to collectively refer to these.

Asana (seat) – a comfortable and steady physical posture of the body.

Ashtanga Yoga (eight-limbed yoga) – the eightfold path of Patanjali.

Atman (Self) – the eternal True Self that can be seen as individual, universal and transcendent (see Brahman and *purusha*).

Avatara – a Divine incarnation, such as Krishna or Shiva.

Avidya (ignorance) – a root cause of suffering (see *vidya*).

Bandha (bond) – locks held by yogis to hold psychic energy in the body.

Bhakta (devotee) – a follower of bhakti yoga.

Bhakti (devotion/love) – devotional yoga towards the Divine or towards a teacher as a manifestation of the Divine.

Bija – literally means 'seed'.

Bindu (point) – the chakra or psychic centre that is seen to be associated with the moon and psychic sounds. Also a source point and centre of energy from which everything was created.

Bodhi (enlightenment) – the state of any enlightened being or Buddha.

Bodhisattva (enlightened being) – in Mahayana Buddhism it is someone who has vowed to put off his or her own final enlightenment in order to help others.

Brahma – one of the personalised Hindu gods. Sometimes seen as the creator and connected with Vishnu as the preserver and Shiva as the destroyer (see *trimurti*).

Brahman – the One Ultimate Reality within and beyond the many forms of the universe (see Nirguna Brahman and Saguna Brahman).

Brahmin – a priest and/or member of the highest social class of traditional Hindu society.

Bramacharya – sexual control. Someone who is celibate.

Buddhi – intuitive and discriminating faculty, which in its highest form, draws upon the consciousness of the *atman*, or in its lowest, categorises sensory information.

Buddha (one who is awake) – someone who is enlightened and has woken up to the truth and is seeing things clearly and as they really are, i.e. as non-separate. Also refers to the historical Buddha who lived and taught around the 5th century bce.

Chakra (wheel) – a principal energy centre in the psychic/subtle body.

Chit (consciousness) – absolute pure Consciousness.

Chitta (that which is conscious) – ordinary individual consciousness (see *antahkarana*). It can be used to describe a variety of mental abilities, including the unconscious mind.

Dharshana (seeing) – a system of Hindu philosophy, or being blessed for being in the sight and presence of a holy person.

Dharma (bearer) – has many meanings, such as 'law', 'righteousness', 'virtue', 'duty' or 'truth', such as the truth of the Buddha's teachings, which one might have first-hand experience and insight into. In orthodox Hinduism, *dharma* is also associated with one's individual duties (*svadharma*) dependent on one's caste.

Dharana (holding) – concentration.

Dhyana (ideation) – a state of meditation.

Diksha (initiation) – being initiated into the practices of yoga.

Duhkha (unsatisfactoriness) – one of three marks of existence in Buddhism.

Ganesha – the elephant headed god of wisdom and remover of obstacles. The son of Shiva and Parvati.

Granthi (knot) – any one of three blockages in the central pathway that prevents full ascent of *kundalini* energy in the psychic body.

Guna (quality) – can mean 'virtue' or any of the three prime qualities of nature
(*prakrti*), such as *tamas* (inertial and/or darkness), *rajas* (acting and dynamic
principle) or *sattva* (purity and/or lucidity).

Guru (teacher) – can refer either to a spiritual teacher who dispels darkness or to
the Divine/God as the supreme Guru.

Hatha Yoga (yoga of force) – a major branch of yoga that places emphasis on
physical postures, cleansing techniques and breathing exercises in order to calm
the mind and exert control over the body.

Ida Nadi (pale conduit) – a psychic passageway in the body. The *prana* current
ascending on the left of the central *shushuma nadi*. Said to have a calming affect
on the mind.

Ishvara (Lord) – refers to either the Creator or a special transient Self (*purusha*).

Ishta – a personal form of God.

Japa (muttering) – the repetition of mantras as forms of meditation.

Jivatman (individual self) – individual 'I' and consciousness, which also has
connections with the Divine as our inner-most being.

Jnana Yoga (yoga of knowledge) – yogic path to freedom via wisdom, discrimination
and intuitive insight.

Kali (the dark one) – a Goddess that displays a destructive aspect.

Kama (desire) – seen as a chief cause of unsatisfactoriness in Hindu yoga and
Buddhism.

Karma (action) – refers to 'actions having consequences' and the will, which
therefore have an effect on one's spiritual progress – in either a positive or
negative way – in this life or a future one. In orthodox Hinduism it is tied-up
with performing one's assigned *dharma*/duty, which is dependent on one's caste.

Karma Yoga (yoga of action) – the path that leads to spiritual liberation through
skilful willed actions.

Kuruna (compassion) – the act of unconditional love for, and empathy with, others.

Kosha (casing/envelope) – any one of the five bodies surrounding the true Self.

Krishna (puller) – an incarnation of the Hindu God Vishnu, who famously
teaches Arjuna about various paths of yoga in the *Bhagavad Gita*.

Khumhaka (pot-like) – breath retention.

Kundalini Shakti (coiled energy) – the manifested spiritual power or serpent
energy that exists in the individual.

Kundalini Yoga (yoga of psychic energy) – a path that seeks liberation through the
use of psychic energy.

Laya Yoga (yoga of dissolution) – a form of Tantra yoga which uses the chakric system and the raising of psychic energy.

Lingam – a symbolic phallus representing Divine creativity – Shiva-*lingam* (see *yoni* and Shiva).

Mahabhutas – the five physical elements of space (or ether), air, fire, water and earth.

Mahat – cosmic intelligence that arose at the creation of the universe.

Mala – beads for counting mantra repetition.

Manas (mind) – the lower functions of the mind and sensory perceptions.

Mandala (circle) – circular design representing the universe and a particular deity.

Mantra Yoga – the repetition of mantras as a path to liberation.

Maya – can have many meanings. In Vedic teachings it referred to creative power in the universe. Later it was associated with an aspect of the goddess and with the world of 'illusion' or 'delusion'.

Moksha (liberation) – freedom from conditioned worldly existence (see *samsara).*

Mooladhara – the chakra which is the seat of sexual and spiritual energy.

Mudra (seal) – a hand or whole body gesture used in mediation.

Nadi (channel) – a passageway for the flow of psychic energy in the body.

Niguna Brahman – Brahman/the Divine in its absolute form, without attributes (see Saguna Brahman).

Nirvana – a state of enlightenment achieved in meditation practices.

Niyama (restraint) – the second limb of Patanjali's *Yoga Sutra* consisting of five inner observances.

Om/Aum – the sacred sound from which the universe was created which symbolises

the Ultimate Reality. It is the highest name of God. The symbol of *Om* represents the individual and Divine consciousness. Its lower curve represent the waking state. The upper curve, dreamless sleep. The curve coming from the middle, the dreaming condition. The semi-circle and dot represent the state of liberation. The repetition of *Om* is said to be a potent sound for awakening to one's spiritual consciousness. It is used in both Tibetan Buddhism and in Hindu yoga.

Patanjali – the compiler of the *Yoga Sutra.*

Parvati (of the mountains) – Shiva's consort and one of many names given to the Divine mother (see *Shakti).*

Pingali Nadi (red conduit) – psychic passageway between the *mooladhara* and *ajna* chakras.

Prajna – consciousness or wisdom.

Prakrti (primal nature) – undifferentiated matter and material of the universe.

Prana – the vital energy in the body and the universal life-force.

Pranayama – the practice of overcoming limitations of the body and mind through the use of psychic and *pranic* energy; particularly with the aid of breathing exercises.

Pratyahara (sensual withdrawal) – withdrawing the mind from distractions.

Purusha – the transcendental pure Self in Samkhya philosophy. In other yoga philosophies it can refer to the higher witness consciousness, the individual spirit and seen as a manifestation of, or comparable to, the *atman*.

Ramanuja – renowned philosopher of 'qualified' non-dualism (1055-1137).

Raga Yoga (Royal Yoga) – another term used for Patanjali's *Yoga Sutra*.

Rig Veda – the oldest of the Vedic/Brahmanical teachings.

Sadhaka – a spiritual seeker.

Sadhana – the term is particularly used in the Tantric tradition and refers to spiritual discipline leading to liberation.

Saguna Brahman – Brahman/the Divine in a personalised form, with qualities and attributes (see Nirguna Brahman).

Sahasrara – the crown chakra and highest energy centre that stands between the psychic and spiritual realms.

Sakshin (the observer) – a non-attached observer consciousness.

Samadhi – the climax of meditation practices where one realises the true Self.

Samkhya – one of the classical schools of Hindu philosophy.

Samsara – the world of conditioned existence in the physical world and bound up with the idea of the continual cycle of lives that people are bound to: birth, death and rebirth.

Samskara (activator) – unconscious imprints and impressions left by volitionary acts which affect our psychological self (see karma).

Sanatana-Dharma – the eternal teaching/truth revealed to the ancient rishis.

Sangha (crowd/host) – a group of students gathered around a teacher. In Buddhism it refers to the community of monks, nuns and lay members.

Sanskrit – the sacred language of the Mahayana Buddhist, Hindu and Jain religions. It is the root language of all European languages.

Santosha – contentment.

Saraswati – a legendary river that is partly underground, which was held as sacred by the people in ancient Vedic times and venerated as a Goddess. Saraswati became the God Brahma's consort. She is seen as the Goddess of scholarship and intuition.

Sat (being/existence) – absolute pure Being.

Shakti (power/force) – the Ultimate Reality in its female aspect, which acts in the universe. Also connected with Kundalini Yoga.

Shankara – (788-820) one of India's greatest philosophers and writers on Advaita Vedanta (non-dualism).

Shiva (the kindly one) – one of the oldest of the Hindu deities that many have speculated to be depicted on ancient seals found in the Indus Valley area (dating back to 2500 bce). He is represented as the *lingam*, has three aspects – creative, preserving and destroying – and seen performing the cosmic dance in the form of Shiva-Nataraja in many statues. He has served *yogins* and *yoginis* throughout the ages and is sometimes placed as part of the *trimurti* along with Vishnu and Brahma as the destroyer.

Shraddha – faith and religious belief.

Shruti (hearing) – revealed sacred teachings of the *Vedas* (see *Vedas* and *Upanishads*).

Siddhi (accomplishment/perfection) – refers to either someone who has accomplished perfection and realised the Absolute or to various psychic powers, including spiritual awakening as the ultimate *siddhi*.

Skandhas (group/aggregate) – term used in Buddhism for the five aggregates that make an individual personality: (1) form, (2) sensations and feelings, (3) conceptions and perception, (4) volition and (5) consciousness.

Smriti (memory) – second category of scared text in Hinduism, such as the *Mahabharata* (which includes the *Bhagavad Gita*), and the *Ramayana*.

Sushuma Nadi (gracious channel) – the central psychic channel or *pranic* current which the serpent energy must ascend to reach the crown chakra in order to achieve liberation.

Sutra (thread) – an aphoristic statement or work containing a collection of statements.

Swadhisthana – the second chakra or psychic centre. It has associations with the unconscious.

Swadhyaya – self-awareness of one's actions and reaction for the purpose of realising one's true Self.

Tanmatras – the five subtle elements of sound, touch, sight, taste and smell.

Tantra (continuity) – refers to Tantra yoga and its teachings which focus on the use of *Shakti* energy.

Tapas (heat) – refers to austerity, which may be done for the purpose of overcoming
> the body and purifying oneself. Was also used to refer to psychic powers in early
> teachings.

Tattva (thatness) – referring to the 'thatness' of a particular reality, such as the ego,
> higher mind or absolute Reality.

Trimurti – three aspects of God that are sometimes shown in the form of Brahma
> the creator, Vishnu the preserver and Shiva the destroyer. It is a popular idea,
> but Hindus and yogis will generally be devoted to just one main God (while
> accepting other manifestations) with more than one aspect to Its nature.

Uma – another form of the Divine Mother and consort of Shiva. She is seen to
> have descended from the Himalayas and is a supreme pinnacle of being, the
> supreme force of the One (see *Parvati* and *Shakti).*

Upanishads (sitting down near) – part of the revealed *Vedic* teachings. Primarily
> mystical teachings that speak from experience of higher states of consciousness,
> the earliest of which dates back to around 800 bce.

Upaya (means) – in Buddhism it is the practice of compassion.

Vandana – prayer.

Vasanas – deep rooted activators in the unconscious mind that inhibit our spiritual
> growth (see *samskara).*

Vedanta (end of the *Vedas*) – one of the six classical systems of Hindu philosophy,
> focusing primarily on the teachings of the *Upanishads, Brahma Sutra* and the
> *Gita* (see Advaita Vedanta, Ramanuja and Shankara).

Vedas – the oldest surviving collection of spiritual and religious teachings of the
> Hindu tradition dating back to around 2500 bce and possibly beyond.

Vidya – knowledge/wisdom (see also *prajna).*

Vishnu – one the most popular gods in the Hindu tradition. Krishna is seen to be
> one of his incarnations.

Vishuddhi – the psychic energy centre or chakra of purification which is centred
> around the throat.

Vritti (whirl) – connected, particularly in Patanjali's *Yoga Sutra,* with
> misconceptions, imagination, cognition, sleep and memory.

Yama (discipline) – the first stage of Patanjali's eight-limbed yoga dealing with
> moral and ethical conduct.

Yantra (devise) – a geometric design that represent one's individual self and a
> particular deity. Used for meditation purposes and realising one's Ultimate

Nature.

Yoga (union/to yoke or to bind) – the unitive discipline of spiritual awakening of which the most popular forms are bhakti, karma and jnana in the Hindu tradition. Yoga is also taught in Buddhism – particularly Tantra yoga in the Tibetan tradition – and Jainism.

Yoga Nidra – a practice of meditation and visualisation known as the 'psychic sleep'.

Yoga Sutra (yogic aphorisms) – compilation of yogic teachings credited to Patanjali around the 2nd century ce. Also known as *Raja Yoga* (Royal Yoga) and 'Classical Yoga': one of the six classical systems of Hindu philosophy.

Yogin – a male student or teacher of yoga.

Yogini – a female student or teacher of yoga.

Yoni (womb) – a symbolic representation of the female sexual organ representing the Creative Mother Energy acting in and beyond the universe (see *lingam*).

Further Reading

An exceptionally important book for today's world.

Universal, transpersonal and integral spirituality

Roberto Assagioli, *Psychosynthesis: A Manual of Principles and Techniques,* Aquarian.

Sri Aurobindo, *A Greater Psychology: An Introduction to the Psychological Thought of Sri Aurobindo* (edited by A.S. Dalal), Tarcher/Putnam.

*Don Edward Beck and Christopher C. Cowan, *Spiral Dynamics: Mastering Values, Leadership and Change,* Blackwell.

*Thomas Berry, *Evening Thoughts: Reflecting on Earth as Sacred Community* (edited by Mary Evelyn Tucker), Sierra Club Books.

Brant Cortright, *Psychotherapy and Spirit: Theory and Practice in Transpersonal Psychotherapy,* SUNY.

Vivianne Crowley, *Jungian Spirituality,* Thorsons.

John Davis, *The Diamond Approach: An Introduction to the Teachings of A. H. Almaas,* Shambhala.

Glyn Edwards and Santoshan, *Tune in to your Spiritual Potential,* Quantum.

Glyn Edwards and Santoshan, *Unleash your Spiritual Power and Grow: Reflect and Learn to Trust the Power Within,* Quantum.

*Matthew Fox, *Creativity: Where the Divine and the Human Meet,* Tarcher/Penguin.

Matthew Fox, *One River, Many Wells: Wisdom Springing from Global Faiths,* Gateway.

*Daniel Goleman (narrated by), *Destructive Emotions and How we can Overcome Them: A Dialogue with the Dalai Lama,* Bloomsbury.

Bede Griffiths, *The One Light: Bede Griffiths Principal Writings* (edited with a commentary by Bruno Barnhart), Templegate.

Christina Grof and Stanislav Grof (edited by), *Spiritual Emergency: When Personal Transformation Becomes a Crisis,* Tarcher/Putnam.

Christina Grof and Stanislav Grof, *The Stormy Search for the Self: Understanding and Living with Spiritual Emergency,* Thorsons.

Jack Kornfield, *After the Ecstasy, the Laundry: How the Heart Grows Wise on the*

Spiritual Path, Rider.

Swami Rama, Rudolph Ballentine and Swami Ajaya, *Yoga and Psychotherapy: The Evolution of Consciousness*, The Himalayan Press.

Indra Sen, *Integral Psychology: The Psychological System of Sri Aurobindo*, Sri Aurobindo Ashram.

Wayne Teasdall, *The Mystic Heart: Discovering a Universal Spirituality in the World's Religions*, New World Library.

Vimala Thakar, *Totality in Essence*, Motilal Banarsidass.

Frank Visser, *Ken Wilber: Thought as Passion*, SUNY.

Joseph Vrinte, *The Quest for the Inner Man: Transpersonal Psychotherapy and Integral Sadhana*, Sri Mira Trust.

Roger Walsh and Frances Vaughan (editors), *Paths Beyond Ego: The Transpersonal Vision*, Tarcher/Putnam.

John Welwood, *Towards a Psychology of Awakening: Buddhism, Psychotherapy, and the Path of Personal and Spiritual Transformation*, Shambhala.

Ken Wilber, *Integral Spirituality: A Startling New Role for Religion in the Modern and Postmodern World*, Integral Books.

The Yogic path

Swami Adiswarananda, *Meditation and its Practices: A Definitive Guide to Techniques and Traditions of Meditation in Yoga and Vedanta*, Skylight Paths.

Sri Aurobindo, *The Integral Yoga: Sri Aurobindo's Teachings and Method of Practice*, Lotus Light.

TKV Desikachar, *Reflections on Yoga Sutras of Patanjali*, Krishnamacharya Yoga Mandiram.

Swami Dharmananda Saraswati, *Breath of Life: Breathing for Health Vitality and Meditation*, Dharma Yoga Centre (and Motilal Banarsidass).

Swami Dharmananda Saraswati, *The Dynamic Body: Movements for Health, Vitality and Holistic Living*, Dharma Yoga Centre (forthcoming).

Mircea Eliade, *Yoga: Immortality and Freedom*, Princeton.

Georg Feuerstein, *The Deeper Dimensions of Yoga: Theory and Practice*, Shambhala.

Georg Feuerstein, *The Shambhala Guide to Yoga*, Shambhala.

Georg Feuerstein, *Tantra: The Path of Ecstasy*, Shambhala.

Julie Friedeberger, *Office Yoga: Tackling Tension with Simple Stretches you can do at your Desk*, Motilal Banarsidass.

B. K. S. Iyengar, *Light on Life: The Journey to Wholeness, Inner Peace and Ultimate*

Freedom, Rodale.

Alan Jacobs, *The Principal Upanishads: A Poetic Translation*, O Books.

Juan Mascaro (translation by), *The Bhagavad Gita*, Penguin Books.

Jugal Kishore Mukherjee, *The Practice of Integral Yoga*, Sri Aurobindo Ashram.

M. P. Pandit, *The Yoga of Self-perfection: Talks Based on Sri Aurobindo's Synthesis of Yoga*, Dipti.

Swami Satyananda Saraswati, *A Systematic Course in the Ancient Tantric Techniques of Yoga and Kriya*, Yoga Publications Trust.

Swami Sivananda Radha: *Mantras: Words of Power*, Timeless Books.

Swami Shankarananda, *Consciousness is Everything: The Yoga of Kashmir Shaivism*, Shaktipat.

The Buddhist path

Ajahn Chah, *Food for the Heart: The Collected Teachings of Ajan Chah*, Wisdom.

Matthew Flickstein, *Swallowing the River Ganges: A Practical Guide to the Path of Purification*, Wisdom.

Ven. Henepola Gunaratana, *Mindfulness in Plain English*, Wisdom.

Thich Nhat Hanh, *The Heart of the Buddha's Teaching: Transforming Suffering into Peace, Joy and Liberation – the Four Noble Truths, the Noble Eightfold Path and other Basic Buddhist Teachings*, Parallax.

Ayya Khema, *Come and See for yourself: The Buddhist Path to Happiness*, Windhorse.

Jack Kornfield, *A Path with Heart: A Guide through the Perils and Promises of Spiritual Life*, Rider.

The Ven. Balangoda Ananda Maitreya (translation by), *The Dhammapada: The Path of Truth* (revised by Rose Kramer), Parallax.

Rob Preece, *The Alchemical Buddha: Introducing the Psychology of Buddhist Tantra*, Mudra Publications.

Walpola Rahula, *What the Buddha Taught*, Oneworld.

Master Sheng-yen with Dan Stevenson, *Hoofprints of the Ox: Principles of the Chan Buddhist Path as Taught by a Modern Chinese Master*, Oxford University Press.

Shunryu Suzuki, *Zen Mind, Beginner's Mind: Informal Talks on Zen Meditation and Practice*, Weatherhill.

Nyanaponika Thera, *The Vision of the Dhamma*, Buddhist Publication Society.

Kosho Uchiyama, *Opening the Hand of Thought: Foundations of Zen Buddhist Practice*, Wisdom.

The Christian path

Alan Jacobs (translated by), *The Gnostic Gospels*, Watkins.

Matthew Fox, *The Coming of the Cosmic Christ*, HarperCollins.

Matthew Fox, *Original Blessing*, Tarcher/Penguin.

Matthew Fox, *Wresting with the Prophets: Essays on Creation Spirituality and Everyday Life*, Tarcher/Putnam.

Joel S. Goldsmith, *Practising the Presence*, Fowler.

Ernest Holmes, *This Thing Called You*, Putnam.

Thomas Keating, *Open Mind, Open Heart: The Contemplative Dimension of the Gospel*, Element.

Ursula King, *Christ in all Things: Exploring Spirituality with Teilhard de Chardin*, SCM Press.

John Main, *Essential Writings* (selected with an introduction by Laurence Freeman), Orbis Books.

Thomas Merton, *New Seeds of Contemplation*, Shambhala.

Henri J. M. Nouwen, *The Only Necessary Things: Living a Prayerful Life* (compiled and edited by Wendy Greer), Darton, Longman and Todd.

John Martin Sahajananda, *You are the Light: Rediscovering the Eastern Jesus*, O Books.

Adrian B. Smith, *The God Shift: Our Changing Perception of the Ultimate Mystery*, Liffey Press.

Brian C. Taylor, *Becoming Human: Core Teachings of Jesus*, Cowley Publications.

Pierre Teilhard de Chardin, *Pierre Teilhard de Chardin* (writings selected with an introduction by Ursula King), Orbis Books.

Influential Jewish writers on philosophy and spirituality

Martin Buber, *I and Thou*, T&T Clark.

Michael Lerner, *Spirit Matters*, Hampton Roads.

Sufi wisdom

James Fadiman and Robert Frager (editors), *Essential Sufism*, Castle.

Llewellyn Vaughan-Lee, *Working with Oneness*, The Golden Sufi Centre.

Spiritual philosophy

S. Abhayananda, *The Wisdom of Vedanta: An Introduction to the Philosophy of Non-dualism*, O Books.

Sri Aurobindo, (compiled with a summary and notes by P. B. Saint-Hilaire), *The Future Evolution of Man: The Divine Life upon Earth (selected from the works of Sri Aurobindo)*, Sri Aurobindo Ashram.

Roy Bhaskar, *Meta-Reality: The Philosophy of meta-Reality, Vol. 1, Creativity, Love and Freedom*, Sage.

Edward Craig (edited by), *The Shorter Routledge Encyclopedia of Philosophy*, Routledge.

Christopher W. Gowans, *Philosophy of the Buddha*, Routledge.

The Dalai Lama (translated and edited by Geshe Thupten Jinpa), *Essence of the Heart Sutra*, Wisdom.

Ian P. McGreal (editor), *Great Thinkers of the Eastern World: The Major Thinkers and Philosophical and Religious Classics of China, India, Japan, Korea and the World of Islam*, HarperCollins.

Swami Prabhavananda and Christopher Isherwood (translated by), *Shankara's Crest-Jewel of Discrimination*, Vedanta Press.

Keith Ward, *Concepts of God: Images of the Divine in Five Religious Traditions*, Oneworld.

Biographies

Shirley Du Boulay, *Beyond the Darkness: A Biography of Bede Griffiths*, O Books.

Shirley Du Boulay, *The Cave of the Heart: The Life of Swami Abhishiktananda*, Orbis.

Ursula King, *Spirit of Fire: The Life and Vision of Teilhard de Chardin*, Orbis Books.

Nyanaponika Thera and Hellmuth Hecker (edited with an introduction by Bhikkhu Bodhi), *Great Disciples of the Buddha: Their Lives, Their Works, Their Legacy*, Wisdom.

Paramahansa Yogananda, *Autobiography of a Yogi*, Self-Realization Fellowship.

For information about the authors visit
www.swamidharmanandasaraswati.com
www.ghf-web.com
www.dharmacentre.org.uk
www.glynedwardscsnu.com

O

is a symbol of the world,
of oneness and unity. O Books
explores the many paths of wholeness and spiritual understanding which
different traditions have developed down
the ages. It aims to bring this knowledge in
accessible form, to a general readership, providing practical spirituality to today's seekers.

For the full list of over 200 titles covering:
ACADEMIC/THEOLOGY • ANGELS • ASTROLOGY/
NUMEROLOGY • BIOGRAPHY/AUTOBIOGRAPHY
• BUDDHISM/ENLIGHTENMENT • BUSINESS/LEADERSHIP/
WISDOM • CELTIC/DRUID/PAGAN • CHANNELLING
• CHRISTIANITY; EARLY • CHRISTIANITY; TRADITIONAL
• CHRISTIANITY; PROGRESSIVE • CHRISTIANITY;
DEVOTIONAL • CHILDREN'S SPIRITUALITY • CHILDREN'S
BIBLE STORIES • CHILDREN'S BOARD/NOVELTY • CREATIVE
SPIRITUALITY • CURRENT AFFAIRS/RELIGIOUS • ECONOMY/
POLITICS/SUSTAINABILITY • ENVIRONMENT/EARTH
• FICTION • GODDESS/FEMININE • HEALTH/FITNESS
• HEALING/REIKI • HINDUISM/ADVAITA/VEDANTA
• HISTORY/ARCHAEOLOGY • HOLISTIC SPIRITUALITY
• INTERFAITH/ECUMENICAL • ISLAM/SUFISM
• JUDAISM/CHRISTIANITY • MEDITATION/PRAYER
• MYSTERY/PARANORMAL • MYSTICISM • MYTHS
• POETRY • RELATIONSHIPS/LOVE • RELIGION/
PHILOSOPHY • SCHOOL TITLES • SCIENCE/
RELIGION • SELF-HELP/PSYCHOLOGY
• SPIRITUAL SEARCH • WORLD
RELIGIONS/SCRIPTURES • YOGA

Please visit our website,
www.O-books.net